Stretch and Strengthen

Stretch

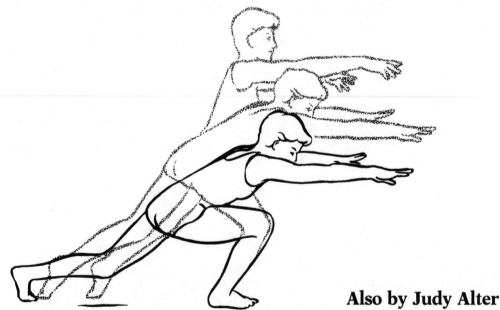

Also by Judy Alter

SURVIVING EXERCISE
Judy Alter's Safe and Sane Exercise Program

and Strengthen

JUDY ALTER

Illustrations by Betsy True

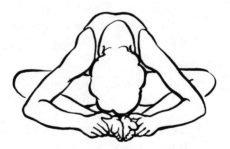

HOUGHTON MIFFLIN COMPANY   BOSTON

To Katherine and Joseph Berkenbilt, my parents, for their loving support and to my many responsive students who asked so many vital questions.

Copyright © 1986 by Judith B. Alter

For information about permission to reproduce selections from this book, write to Permissions, Houghton Mifflin Company, 215 Park Avenue South, New York, New York 10003.

Library of Congress Cataloging-in-Publication Data

Alter, Judy.
  Stretch and strengthen.
  1. Exercise.   2. Stretch (Physiology).   3. Muscle strength. I. Title.
  RA781.63.A47   1986   613.7'1   85-21975
  ISBN 0-395-36263-6
  ISBN 0-395-52808-9 (pbk.)

Printed in the United States of America

CRS 10 9 8 7 6

Acknowledgments

These words touch only the surface of the gratitude that I feel to the many people who helped immeasurably to bring this book from its inception to its completed form. There is not enough space here to list the names of my students whose questions stimulated the discovery of some of the most powerful exercises in this book. Nor is there space to list the names of my dance colleagues who encouraged me to write down my stretch-strengthen system.

I want to thank Betsy True for photographing and drawing the illustrations with such painstaking care and devotion; Patricia Foley for patiently modeling for the illustrations; Judy Sidran and Al Berman for commenting on early versions of the manuscript; and René Cailliet, M.D., for his supportive comments and helpful suggestions.

I am also grateful to Austin Olney, director of trade publishing of Houghton Mifflin, for urging me to complete this book; Lisa Bennett, whose early guidance about getting this manuscript published enabled me to secure Houghton Mifflin as my publisher; Ruth Hapgood, my editor and friend, who believes so strongly in these exercises, for wisely, patiently, and brilliantly helping me put these exercises into words, these ideas into logical sequence, and the material into a meaningful whole; Janet Silver for editing the manuscript with the skill of a detective and the wisdom of a symbolic logician; Copenhaver Cumpston for artistically and accurately designing the pages and weaving the words and pictures together; and Bernard and Nan Locker for persuading me to buy a word processor.

To the students of the Loretto Heights College (Denver, Colorado) Ballet Institute, 1985, an extra word of appreciation for helping me figure out some vital details I had not previously discovered. I must thank Jenny Hunter, outstanding dancer, choreographer, and teacher, for stimulating my inventiveness and specifically for Hiccup and Pretzel.

Author's Note

This book contains methods of exercise that I have found effective through my personal experience in working with students and in rehabilitating private clients. My recommendations are not meant to substitute for medical advice. I suggest exercises to lessen and eliminate pain and soreness, but these are not substitutes for medical procedures.

We all deal with the ordinary aches and pains of exercise, but if you have any other physical condition that concerns you, you need to sort it out with your doctor before undertaking any form of exercise.

In particular, throughout the rehabilitation section of this book, I repeatedly emphasize that medical doctors should be consulted about trying what I counsel.

Some of the people I have worked with have been referred to me by physicians, and I have helped some physicians themselves. I have written this book out of my experience of the usefulness of these forms of exercise, but it should be clear that this is not medical treatment.

Contents

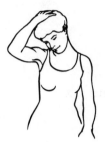
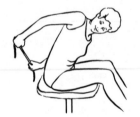

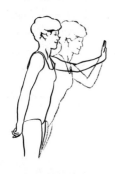
Chapter 7

Your Wrists, Hands, and Fingers   74

Anatomy   74

EXERCISES

Chapter 8

Your Rib Cage   83

Anatomy   83

EXERCISES

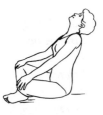
Chapter 9

Your Abdominal Muscles   91

Anatomy   91

EXERCISES

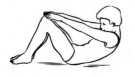
Chapter 10

Your Lower Back and Hips   102

Anatomy   102

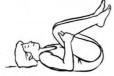

EXERCISES

Chapter 11

Your Thighs: Front and Back   121

Anatomy   121

EXERCISES

Chapter 12

Your Thighs: Inner and Outer   143

EXERCISES

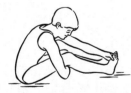

Chapter 13

Your Lower Leg   164

Anatomy   164

EXERCISES

Chapter 14

Your Feet   174

Anatomy   174

EXERCISES

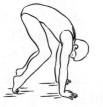

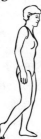

Chapter 15

Chapter 16

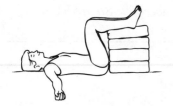

Foreword

Exercise books may come and go but exercise methods that are as revolutionary as Judy Alter's will surely have an impact for years to come. Her method of stretching and strengthening will prove to be not only the treatment but also the cure for many of our muscle aches and pains. The medical establishment is often accused — and rightly so — of concentrating too much on treating maladies and not enough on finding their causes. It is rare to find both prevention and cure in the same package, but that's exactly what Judy Alter has come up with.

The Alter method answers numerous questions that many of us have had about the value of the warm-up in an exercise program. Until this book, the whole concept of stretching and strengthening — both the method of doing it and the reason for doing it — has been poorly defined. One result has been that too many people have suffered injuries from jumping into their exercise programs too quickly. However, by combining a strengthening routine with stretching, you can make this "golden period" as important as it really is. It is absolutely the key to a well-balanced body and a well-balanced exercise program. Whether you are a dancer or jogger, amateur or professional, efficient strengthening and stretching without overtightening is essential.

Unlike any other exercise or therapy book that I have come across, the Alter method shows in exact detail how to perform each exercise and how that exercise relates to a specific problem. Whether it is shin splints or back pain, she shows how to correct it. She divides the torso into parts and then shows how to exercise each part correctly and effectively. Then she joins all of these parts together, devising a method that applies to everybody, from the beginner to the professional.

I have found the Alter stretch method particularly useful

in my practice. Patients who have come to me with tennis elbow, low-back pain, sciatica, and shin splints have all profited from her method. These are people who have already tried drug therapy, steroid injections, and pain killers. Her exercises have allowed them to go back to their jobs and their sports activities without pain and without drugs.

On a personal level I have found her program even more important. Last year my wife, Penelope, was in an automobile accident that resulted in a terribly debilitating whiplash injury. We have three children and a very full schedule, and our whole family was in despair. Penelope tried everything from arthritis medications to physical therapy, from acupuncture to calcium tablets. Being a physician, I was able to obtain the finest medical care available, but to no avail. That's where Judy Alter came in. From the eventful day that we met her at the home of our friends, Ben and Judy Sidran (Judy has been an active student of Ms. Alter's for several years), Penelope's pain began to diminish and her rehabilitation commenced. To this day Penelope has continued to follow the Alter stretch method on a regular basis, and she remains pain free.

Virtually everyone who exercises or has had painful muscles can benefit from following the activities outlined in this book. Judy Alter disproves the "no pain, no gain" theory time and time again. She explains the stretch reflex in detail and outlines a cure for what we physicians call "soft tissue arthritis," or those painful muscles that are thought to account for 25 percent of all visits to physicians for arthritis.

Sometimes what is obvious is the most difficult to discover. Judy Alter's methods seem so obvious and natural once you have tried them that you cannot understand why you haven't used them before. But once you do, you will feel so much better that going back to your old routine will become out of the question.

Robert (Zorba) Paster, M.D.
Assistant Clinical Professor,
University of Wisconsin Medical School,
Madison, Wisconsin

Introduction: This Book Is Different

The exercise system in this book combines a new method of stretching your muscles with the most efficient way to strengthen them. To keep your body in motion, you need to balance the use of your muscles by stretching the ones you strengthen and strengthening the ones you stretch. The stretch and strengthen system presented here has been developed to do just that, so that increasing your muscles' strength will not make them overtight, and stretching will not make them weak or vulnerable. The exercises also help you heal injured muscles and safely mobilize unused or weak ones.

This new method for stretching your muscles is a major advance over other methods used today. So if you want to be able to stretch your muscles 10 to 12 inches farther in the most common stretch positions and not be sore tomorrow, the exercises in this book will help you to do this.

This new stretch system is combined with the most recent knowledge about strengthening your muscles. Do you want a slimmer waistline, thinner thighs, and firmer, stronger arms? Do you want to get rid of a double chin, round shoulders, or "love handles"? The strengthening exercises here can help you.

Look through the book. You will see that the pictures of the exercises look different from the ones you are currently doing (unless you are already doing the exercises in my earlier book, *Surviving Exercise* [Boston: Houghton Mifflin, 1983]). They *are* different. They are carefully worked out so that you stretch your muscles or strengthen them. And the positions enable you to stretch or strengthen only your muscles, not your ligaments, so you should experience no "Ouch!" pain, little discomfort, and no injury.

These exercises feel different because they either relax the muscles you are stretching or tire and warm the muscles you are strengthening. The "feel" of the exercise actually guides you while you do the exercises, and that itself is different. And while the exercises don't give you a "burn," they actually work!

The exercises also help you to recover from injury. Do you suffer from shin splints, tendinitis, fallen arches, or a sore neck? You've come to the right place because *Stretch and Strengthen* explains how to recover from many common injuries that derive from your own special body structure and overuse or misuse of your moving parts.

This is a how-to book for your muscles: how to safely *stretch* the muscles that you strengthen and tighten in your daily, recreational, fitness, and sports activities; and how to sanely *strengthen* the muscles that your activities stretch. You can learn how to stretch and strengthen your muscles safely and sanely and in that way keep them mobile. By moving your muscles properly, you'll develop muscles that will keep your body in motion.

For years people doing and teaching exercise never questioned whether or not the exercises actually worked. Now there are specialists studying the results of a wide variety of activities. This book applies information from the fields of anatomy, kinesiology, exercise physiology, physical therapy, sports medicine, and rehabilitation medicine. The exercises have also been used by thousands of people, in dance classes, sports activities, and exercise workshops. The exercises correct, rearrange, or reinvent many of the common ones so that they actually give you the results you want.

The Alter Stretch Method presented here originally was introduced in *Surviving Exercise*. Now you can understand how it works and learn thirty-eight safe and sane stretching exercises. *Stretch and Strengthen* uses isotonic strengthening exercises and explains how and why this method is so effective for building basic strength in your muscles as well as endurance and power. You can also learn to do forty-three strengthening exercises that work, are efficient, and don't make your muscles sore. Chapter 3 outlines a variety of exercise programs to use in getting ready to do most daily chores and popular recreational, fitness, and sports activities. Chapter 15 offers you guidelines for standing correctly aligned and for balancing, walking, running, and jumping. And the last chapter offers you guidelines for taking special care of your body.

Since it is so hard to learn exercises from a book, the exercise chapters are designed to help you overcome this difficulty. Each chapter has two sections. The first is a simple anatomical description of the bones, range of movement, and muscles of each major area of your body. The anatomy description is there to help you understand why and how the exercises work. The second section contains lots of stretching and strengthening exercises. In several chapters, there is a *readying position* to help you align your whole body while you concentrate on one particular body part.

Each exercise gives a *starting position*, which tells you how to arrange your body before you begin the exercise. The steps of each exercise are then described in detail and given suggested counts. Throughout, there are *troubleshooting* notes to keep you from making mistakes.

And there are two kinds of pictures. The pictures for the stretching exercises show only the positions in which you hold your body. That is because to stretch muscles adequately, you need to *hold positions for at least 30 seconds to a minute*. The pictures for the strengthening exercises indicate movement, not holding, to show how you should *move your body slowly down and up against gravity*. All the pictures show the exact correct position described in the text. There are only a few pictures to show you what *not* to do.

The exercises have evolved over fifteen years and have been done by thousands of people — old and young, professional and amateur — in dance classes and exercise workshops across the country. Instructions for the exercises use words that seem to help many people learn how to do them precisely and correctly.

Glossary

The terms below are listed in order of their importance, so they are not alphabetical.

Stretch: The elastic characteristic of muscle tissue. Muscle tissue is like a rubber band: when you lengthen muscles, they expand and extend; when you release the pull, they contract back to their resting length. See Chapter 2.

Strength: The property of muscle that lets you lift, carry, hold, push, pull, and do other kinds of work. Muscles get strong and do their jobs because they contract and shorten. In that way they pull your bones together. See Chapter 2.

Active: This term is very important for your understanding of how to use this book. When you exercise, you can simply move your limbs around with a minimum of energy. That is the opposite of active: that is passive. Or you can move your body parts in space with energy and deliberate intention so that they cut through space the way a knife cuts through cheese. That is active and that is the way these exercises should be done. When the instructions say to pull your head down to your feet, you should use your arm muscles energetically to pull your upper body down to your feet. Really pull — steadily and carefully, but really pull. Such pulling is an example of "active" stretching. See Chapter 2.

Feel: This term is also very important. You need to constantly monitor the sensations going on in your muscles. You want to *feel* the stretching or strengthening all along the *surface* of the muscles you are using, not at a specific *point* in the joint. See Chapter 2 for details about distinguishing among the sensations of stretching, strengthening, and pain.

Arch: What you do *not* want to do with your lower back and neck. You arch when you bend your upper body backward with your head aiming toward your heels. Back bends in gymnastics arch your back. Head circles arch your neck. These movements can permanently damage the discs in your spine. See the anatomy section in Chapter 10.

Bounce: A percussive way that some people still mistakenly use to stretch their muscles. Because bouncing is a stretch followed by a contraction, one right after the other, the one cancels out the effectiveness of the other, so bouncing is useless! It is a major cause of soreness in your muscles, which is unnecessary when you exercise.

Click or **Pop:** The unpleasant sound and feeling of tendons or ligaments rolling over each other or snapping bones back into place. Doing a lot of exercises that produce this sound can irritate your tissues and may cause "wear and tear" arthritis. You can avoid this sensation by moving your body parts slowly and finding a way to prevent the discomfort and misalignment from occurring. See Chapters 15 and 16.

Lock: What happens when you overzealously extend your arms or legs so that you are pressing the bones in your joints to the joints' most extreme tautness. If you have loose ligaments, your knees and elbows can even bend back beyond their straight, extended position. That is called hyperextension. When you lock, you can feel the sensation of grinding bone on bone in your joints and an uncomfortable tightness in your ligaments. When you relax and take away the grinding and tight sensations, you have merely straightened your legs and arms and they are no longer locked. Locking permanently stretches ligaments that, like leather, can stretch but not contract back to their original length, and it can really irritate your bones. You can and should learn never to lock your joints.

Overbend: The equally harmful opposite of lock: folding your knees, elbows, and neck too much. This can happen when you sit directly on top of your lower legs, do deep knee bends incorrectly, do a shoulder stand, or go too low doing push-ups. You have no muscle control when you let your arms or legs fold too much. Overbending, like locking, stretches your ligaments, which don't contract; it can make the cartilage between your bones more vulnerable to tearing; and it can make your muscles more susceptible to strains and tears. Don't let it happen when exercising or any other time.

Swing: What your arms do naturally as a result of momentum when you walk or run. Swinging exercises do not stretch or strengthen your muscles because they use your muscles passively and depend only on movement in your joints, with your limbs hanging on your ligaments.

Slowly: Seconds on the clock are slow enough for you to use in the exercises in which the instructions say "slowly." At first you may need extra patience to do strengthening exercises slowly, but soon you will see how effective doing these exercises slowly is. Then you may want to move even more slowly.

Warm-up: Ask five people what they mean by warm-up and you will get five different answers. The experts agree only that before you exercise you need to raise your core (internal) body temperature from its resting state (what it is when you get out of bed in the morning). The experts also say not to do any stretching exercises unless your muscles are "warm," that is, slightly soft or more gelatinous. (Muscles, tendons, and ligaments are like gelatin. When you put gelatin on the stove, it melts; in the refrigerator, it hardens.) Most of the popular ways of stretching are ineffective. The stretching exercises shown here are effective and cause no soreness or injury. You should be up and out of bed for about 20 minutes before you start any exercise. Then your internal temperature and muscles are warm enough to begin the stretching exercises.

*

There is a lot of material here and you can use it in lots of ways. Use it as a whole or in parts; for separate parts of your body or for your entire body; or just for rehabilitation. Use it to learn how to do the exercises or for the information you can get about how and why your body works the way it does. But, however you do, do use it.

1

The Function of Exercise in Sports and Dance

Why, you ask, is it important to clarify the function of exercise in sports and dance? Everyone knows that activities like baseball, basketball, soccer, and ballet have always had special exercises that help you train for these activities. And when you decide to learn how to do ballet or play baseball or tennis you accept these training techniques and trust that they will help you dance or play your sport with ease and coordination. Even the simplest and most popular activities, such as jogging and disco dancing, have warm-up exercises and special techniques to enable you to enjoy and increase your skill. So far, this all seems obvious and sensible: the exercises you do to learn and to increase your ability in sports and dance come from the activity itself and its specific demands on your body. That seems okay, doesn't it?

But shouldn't these techniques come from you, the person doing the activity, and shouldn't they fit the limits and range of your unique body? You say, "Yes, they should, but I'm just a beginner and I don't know how to make my body do all those fancy moves and strenuous coordinations. Experts who know how to do those things should work out the ways to help me learn how." But experts already know how to play or dance; and they have, inadvertently, already adapted the exercises and activities to their own experi-

1

enced and coordinated bodies. Often it has been a long time since those experts were beginners.

"But," you might say, "it is important to have techniques fit each physical activity people want to learn. And isn't it the purpose of these techniques to solve the movement problems inherent in each activity?" Yes, they should and often do. For example, in order to jump and land properly, dancers do a sequence of techniques known as pliés and relevés. This means you bend your knees, keeping your heels on the floor (plié); then straighten your knees, lift your heels, and rise directly on the balls of your feet and toes (relevé); and finally sink down again to a standing position by replacing your heels on the floor. If done properly (see Chapter 13), this sequence should increase your ankle flexibility and calf and toe strength, should help you practice proper leg alignment, and should enable you to use your legs and feet effectively and efficiently to jump buoyantly.

Fine, no problem here. But is there? This technique assumes toe strength, ankle and knee alignment, and Achilles tendon flexibility, as well as proper placement of the rest of the body. Not all beginners have this. This technique also assumes that you have "normal" joint range, not extra-long ligaments and too flexible joints (or tight ligaments and inflexible joints). Pliés and relevés are often done to music, which again puts the activity first, not the needs of people with varying strength and flexibility, body awareness, placement, and experience. Besides, in a real leap you jump from bent knees and land with them bent, so by practicing this sequence of movements (straightening your legs before you lift your heels up), you are practicing the exact opposite of the correct use of your legs. Dancers continue to do these exercises this way because that is the tradition.

If you are like most people, when you begin to learn an activity, you simply assume that you will work to fit your body into the mold that the training methods demand. You expect to train until your body fits the needs and style of your activity. This is *backward* and a major cause of injury. Injuries often occur when techniques are not anatomically balanced or wise. Injuries can occur because teachers and coaches are often unable to explain how to execute the technique or even why it is done. Your body may become more prone to injury because you have been allowed to carry out the techniques incorrectly. Sometimes you appear to be doing them correctly, but you really feel discomfort and out-and-out pain and don't say so. Finally, injuries can occur because your muscles have not been readied by proper stretching and strengthening for the specialized exercises you are being asked to do.

Some exercise systems derive from ancient practices, and their followers believe unquestioningly in their value. Proponents of yoga and gymnastics often cite long tradition as a reason to continue using the entire system even when some of the exercises are known to produce serious injury. "Look at my teacher!" is a common argument. Teachers and outstanding figures in these fields are often cited as examples of excellent health and longevity to show that the systems do not cause debilitating injury. There is no way to prove that these people might also be in excellent health and long-lived without the yoga or gymnastics. What is ignored is the unknown number of once-active teachers, leaders, and students who have suffered disabling injury from these exercise practices.

Furthermore, hereditary and cultural factors contribute to the unusual success of leaders in specialized activities like yoga and gymnastics. People in twentieth-century America may not have inherited the body type or live in a manner that enables them to participate easily in these activities and come away with the same benefits. Some examples will make this idea clear. In Oriental cultures, instead of sitting on chairs, it is common to work or hold conversations in a deep squatting position, with the entire foot flat on the floor, knees pointing directly up, and with the hips and torso comfortably close to the thighs. The shape of the body in this sitting position is like an N. Frequently these people also sit or kneel directly on the lower legs, with the feet uncurled and with the weight of the hips resting on the feet. (Imagine a flattened Z.) In countries where these squatting and kneeling positions are common, the traditional clothing covers the legs in a manner that allows people to be comfortable.

The squatting position is anatomically sound because the body weight is placed directly on the whole foot and is suspended on upright lower leg bones; that is, the weight is held by bones. In our society, when people squat, their weight is often only on their toes. The lower leg bone is on a diagonal. In this position, then, the ligaments of the knee, which attach the thigh bone to the lower leg, are bearing the entire body weight and so this semisquatting position can cause considerable strain on the knee joint. The Oriental squat requires and maintains a flexible Achilles tendon, at the base of the heel; people in Western society, who do not commonly use this posture and who wear shoes with heels, tend to have less flexible Achilles tendons. This deep squatting position is, therefore, uncomfortable for many Westerners who do not have loose ligaments. There are also physical consequences for the knees of people who frequently use the deep squat and kneeling sitting positions. People who use these postures have wider knees than those of people in cultures where chairs, heeled shoes, and displayed legs are valued.

The lotus sitting position in yoga is most easily done by people whose bodies have flexible hip joints. Joint flexibility is usually due to the length of the ligaments that hold the bones together. Hypermobility (misnamed "double-jointedness") is a hereditary characteristic. Yoga and gymnastics were developed by people for whom these positions and strenuous moves were easy. Many of the positions and moves in these activities can permanently harm people with a "normal" range of motion in their joints.

Hereditary hypermobility contributes to the "natural selection" of dancers, gymnasts, and people who are good at yoga. In England, a study was made of the inherited flexibility of fifty-three students at the Royal School of Ballet and their families. For a control group, the study tested nursing students of similar age and height. Both groups were examined for range of flexibility in six joints. The mobility of the fifth finger (the little finger) was almost the same in both groups. (This joint served as a control measure.) In the other areas of the body where hypermobility is common, namely the thumb, elbow, knee, ankle, and spine, the ballet students had a range twice or more as great as the nursing students. This "natural selection" probably occurs when these flexible-jointed people are young. Their range of motion becomes apparent early and they are encouraged to go into activities like dance or gymnastics.

Although highly skilled, physically demanding activities such as ballet, yoga, and gymnastics have traditionally capitalized on hypermobility, the permanent injury and pain associated with these activities has been constant, though little public notice has been taken. Dr. James A. Nicholas, founder and editor of the *American Journal of Sports Medicine*, urges that boys and men in high school and college sports be screened for hypermobile joints, especially the knee. He feels that those with hypermobile knees should *not* be allowed to participate in injury-producing games such as football and basketball; the documented rate of injury in football players with hypermobile knees is 70 percent higher than those with a "normal" range.

Indeed, pain and persistent disability are often taken for granted when young people participate in these activities. Youthful participation in acrobatics and ballet for women, and high school and college sports for men, probably has been a major contributing cause of bad knees and severe back pain in many adults from the middle years on. This cause has often been overlooked by physicians. Low back pain is a common complaint among at least 80 percent of adult Americans. There are many causes for this (see Chapter 16), not the least of which are poor posture, locked knees, uneven leg length, poor abdominal muscle tone, and incorrect or ineffective exercise done in the name of fitness or in preparation for playing a game.

Most people these days know how important it is to be physically active. The positive effects — burning calories, toning muscles, reducing stress, and increasing one's sense of well-being — are well publicized. There are now thirty million Americans jogging and probably as many people exercising in aerobics and fitness classes. The negative results of these active pastimes are handled by physicians in a new field, sports medicine. This specialty has developed along with the fitness craze to handle the epidemic of injuries. Publicity is now given to the pain, strain, and personal sacrifice of the many people who have to drop out of their sports or dance activity because of injury. In an article entitled "Can Aerobics Endanger Your Fitness?"(*Boston Globe*,

February 18, 1983), Karen S. Peterson wrote: "No federal agency logs statistics associated with dance/exercise injuries. But the sense of those within the industry who are deeply troubled is that aerobic dance classes are producing a small army of the walking wounded." This level of injury is probably as high from the current weight-lifting craze as well. "Sports medicine experts generally agree that nearly 80 percent of all recreational injuries are preventable and can probably be avoided through intelligent stretching" (*Your Health and Fitness* 5, no. 4, August/September 1983). Traditional forms of stretching and strengthening that derive from the activities themselves are not necessarily intelligent, and since few coaches and teachers are trained in anatomy and kinesiology, safe and sane ways of stretching and strengthening are not widely used in tradition-bound sports and dance activities.

This book contains a series of stretching and strengthening exercises that can prepare your muscles for any physical activity. If your muscles are ready, you can prevent undue stress on your ligaments and joints. These exercises are effective for tight-, normal-, and loose-ligamented people. The exercises capitalize on and synthesize the most pertinent information gathered from research in the fields of anatomy, kinesiology, neuroanatomy, and exercise physiology. Using these exercises, it is possible for you to prevent severe bodily injuries in most physically demanding activities. (See *Surviving Exercise*, for the exercises and positions *not* to do.) These training techniques are based on the body's muscular power and its joints' range of motion. The exercises will enable you to fit the activities of your choice to your adequately stretched and strengthened body.

2 Principles of Stretching and Strengthening

Body Basics

All the physical activity that you do happens because your muscles move. To say this another way, your moving muscles move you. This simple but important idea needs some explanation. Before you can make sense of this chapter's principles of stretching and strengthening, you need some information about the structure of your body and how it moves.

Bones: Your skeleton consists of 206 bones, which in concert support your body. They are your framework; they are rigid and are not meant to bend. They cannot move by themselves.

Joints: Joints are where your bones connect. The directions in which your various bones can move are determined by the shape of the bones where they meet. The range of motion in each joint is determined by the looseness or tightness of your ligaments and the stretchiness and strength of your muscles.

Ligaments: Ligaments hold the bones together at the joints. Ligaments are pliable, but they are not elastic. They permit or restrict the bones' movement in the same way that a hinge functions on a door. Ligaments do not contract or move on their own and once they are stretched, like leather, they don't unstretch.

Muscles: Muscles contract to move your bones at their joints — that's the miracle of movement. Muscles are elastic, and they move your bones because they shorten. They are located in sets on opposite sides of bones. When the muscles on one side of a bone shorten, the muscles on the other side lengthen. To see how this works, bend your hand forward at the wrist. The muscles on the palm side of your forearm shorten, and the muscles on the top of your wrist and forearm lengthen. The active part of the muscle action is the shortening, the contraction, which in turn lengthens or stretches the opposite set. You initiate the muscle action from a stretched or relaxed position.

Tendons: Tendons are the harder, narrower ends of muscles that attach the muscles to the bones. Tendons are very much like ligaments: they are pliable but not elastic. Tendons connect muscles to bones, and ligments connect bones to other bones.

*

So, muscles are the moving force of your body. The force of a muscle is transmitted to the bones by the tendons. Your brain thinks a movement; your nerves carry the message to your muscles; and your muscles move your bones. Except where gravity pulls part of the body passively, movement almost always involves the contraction of some muscles and the stretching of others. This changes the position of the bones, which move at the joints.

Guidelines for Using Your Muscles

Your muscles must be strong and they must also be elastic and able to stretch so they can do anything you want them to do. Daily activity does not provide your muscles with a balance of stretching and strengthening; even walking, sitting, and sleeping unevenly stretch some muscles and tighten others. That is why you are told to stretch before and after most strenuous activity.

Six guidelines can enable you to protect your body in any exercise situation.

1. Be guided by the inherited and developed limits of your body.
2. As a mode of living, *keep moving*, because for muscles to be useful, they must be used.
3. *Feel* all muscle activity when you are exercising to get ready to do physical activity. Trust your perception of muscles relaxing (stretching) and contracting (strengthening).
4. *Stop* any and all activity if it hurts — "Ouch!" hurts.
5. *Strengthen* the muscles that you have stretched or will stretch.
6. Before and after any activity, *stretch* the muscles that the activity strengthens.

Be guided by the inherited and developed limits of your body. You inherit tight, loose, or "normal" ligaments, and this structure cannot be changed, though it can be modified and adapted to activity. Often people with loose ligaments (incorrectly called double-jointed) think they don't need to stretch any of their muscles, and if they do try stretching, they often don't feel the stretches in their muscles.

People with tight ligaments are much less prone to joint injury, but they often experience discomfort in their joints during exercise because when unstretched muscles are stretched incorrectly they will create a strong stretch sensation across the joints as well as in the muscles. Both tight- and loose-ligamented people need to understand their bodies' natural limits and to adapt their activity accordingly.

Keep moving: to be useful, muscles must be used. Inadequately stretched and strengthened muscles are not very useful, and entirely unused muscles atrophy; that is, they shrink in size and lose their ability to contract with power or relax (stretch) from their contraction.

Recent medical practice recognizes the healthy results of exercise; in fact, doctors now instruct their surgery patients to get up and walk as soon as possible, usually within 24 hours after an operation. The recovery is faster if a patient's

how to determine?

entire body is kept active. This idea is true for most injuries. Motion is healing. See Chapter 16 for more information about recovering from injury.

Feel all exercises in your muscles and learn to trust your perception of strength and stretch sensations. When you exercise for strength or stretch, you should experience the sensations in your muscles. The release of tension that stretching produces is a strong and satisfying sensation in your muscles. *Correct stretching requires that you hold your position until the tension in the muscle releases. This usually takes about a minute*, though you may need to hold a position longer to feel the tightness of the muscle release. And you know the sensation of muscles strengthening from the fatigue of bearing a weight, for instance, after carrying a heavy bag of groceries up several flights of stairs. *Correct strengthening involves working muscles slowly, up and down against gravity, just a little beyond their point of fatigue.* When you stop the stretching or strengthening activity, the sensations should go away fairly soon without residual burning or tightness.

Stop any and all activity if it hurts — "Ouch!" hurts. You know the feeling of "ouch!" pain. It stings, it is hot, it makes you jump or cringe or suddenly cry out. "Ouch!" pain can be a life-saving signal and should not be endured. During exercise, feelings of muscle contraction (the exertion from strengthening) and the release of tension from stretching are safe. The sensation of "ouch!" is a signal to **STOP!**

See *Surviving Exercise* for details about unsafe exercises. Some excess discomfort or strong twinges may come from your doing an exercise that is too hard for your inadequately toned muscles, and sometimes pain can result from strain on already injured areas of your body. In any case, if you feel "ouch!" pain, **ALWAYS STOP!**

Some exercises do not feel painful when you're doing them, but pain or injury may surface one or two days later. For example, bouncing, swinging, or doing strengthening exercises too fast can often cause day-after soreness. Another kind of pain can come about from a fall, a sudden and unexpected move, or lifting or carrying an exceptionally heavy object. These types of injuries are harder to prevent but their pain can be minimized if you do proper warm-up and cool-down exercises.

Exercises should not make your muscles sore and aching, and if done correctly they should be satisfying enough in themselves to keep you doing them. The exercises in this book should produce little lasting soreness.

Strengthen the muscles you stretch. Three areas of your body need careful strengthening because daily activities and recreational exercise do not automatically do the job: your abdominal muscles (see Chapter 9), the back of your shoulders (see Chapter 5), and the front of your neck (see Chapter 4).

Stretch the muscles you strengthen. Muscles don't stretch on their own. Make a fist and hold the contraction for 30 seconds. Now stop making a fist and just relax your grip. What happens? On their own, your fingers don't uncurl or stretch out. You have to do that as a separate action. In order for your muscles to contract, they need to start in a relaxed or stretched position. You always need to balance stretching with strengthening, and strengthening with correct and adequate stretching.

The Alter Method of Stretching

Now that you understand why your muscles must have a balance of stretching and strengthening activity to keep them toned and useful, you are ready to turn your mind and body to the Alter Method of Stretching. It has six features: traction, contraction, action, separation, relaxation, and sensation.

Traction: This stretch method works the way traction does. When muscles are in a severe contracture, which is like a muscle cramp multiplied by ten (very painful!), an orthopedist often applies traction to eliminate the pain. The doctor will hang weights from the part of the body that is in contracture. The weight simply tires the muscles so they relax, let go, and lengthen. With this lengthening, the pain stops. Sometimes this procedure takes only a few hours.

The Alter Method of Stretching positions parts of your

11

body in such a way as to use their own inherent weight to tire the muscles to be stretched. For instance, your head weighs 10 to 12 pounds. When it hangs down in the correct hamstring-stretch position, its weight helps fatigue the hamstrings and so they relax and stretch more easily (see Chapter 11). This hanging also relaxes some of your neck muscles. (This idea is not new. Carol J. Widule states this principle in her chapter "Conditioning" in *Introduction to Human Movement,* edited by Hope M. Smith [Reading, Mass.: Addison-Wesley, 1968].)

Contraction: Another way this method tires the muscles to be stretched is by using them to lift and lower a limb or body part. When lifting and lowering, your muscles are contracting, which strengthens them. When your muscles are tired from lifting and lowering, they also relax and lengthen more easily. You derive a double benefit from this part of the process, since even while taking the time to stretch your muscles, you are often strengthening them. The strengthening activity happens before or after holding muscles in a stretching position, not simultaneously.

As one of its several elements, this method uses a built-in body reflex that is variously known as the stretch reflex, reciprocal innervation, reciprocal inhibition, or PNF (proprioceptor neuromuscular facilitation). Simply stated, when one group of muscles is called on to work very hard or very quickly, the opposite set of muscles relaxes to enable the moving muscles to do their job. Part of this process is reflexive, or automatic. You have experienced this reflex when you suddenly withdraw your hand from a fire or a hot handle. In the stretch system called PNF, this reflex is used to help stretch muscles with isometric (holding) and then isotonic (moving) contractions and involves a partner. Without using a partner, the Alter Method of Stretching uses this physiologically automatic mechanism; namely, muscles stretch more easily after their opposites have been contracting. The contractions can be either isometric (static and holding) or isotonic (moving down and up against the pull of gravity).

Action: A third part of this method has you actively stretch your muscles. Remember, muscles are elastic, like rubber bands. When you are doing one of the stretching exercises, the instructions will often tell you to use your arm strength to actively pull one part of your body down or toward another part of your body, or to hug with your arms to hold your chest and pelvis "glued" to your thigh, as in the Hamstring Stretch (exercise 71). Active stretching is just as safe as passive stretching, where you let your upper body hang down without pulsing or bouncing. Passive stretching is much safer than percussive or ballistic stretching, such as bouncing. Bouncing is forceful and can tear the cross fibers that hold your muscle fibers together, because half of the bounce action is a contraction. The Alter Method goes beyond passive stretching because it uses muscles of other parts of your body (often your arms) to actively pull instead of waiting to have the stretch occur on its own. This active stretching does not cause soreness or injury because the stretching muscles themselves are only lengthening. The position of the other body parts is specified because their weight assists in lengthening the stretching muscles.

Separation: The Alter Method works with one part of your body at a time. Instead of stretching both calf muscles at the same time, you stretch one leg and then the other. The same is true for all the other parts of your body. It is easier to concentrate on the right "feel" of one part at a time. And you can much more easily endure the initial discomfort of starting to stretch tight muscles when you separate your body into parts and stretch them singly. Your ability to endure the feeling of tightness as it relaxes will be assisted by the next part of the stretching method, relaxation.

Relaxation: You can teach yourself to relax on command by practicing any one of the several relaxation techniques that have been developed. They all involve your learning to feel tension in your muscles and then learning to let it go. Your first natural response to any sensation, even to the sensation of stretching your muscles, is likely to be one of tightening up, if only a little. So you need to be aware that your body will respond in a way that can temporarily inhibit the stretching that you set out to do. When you feel yourself tightening up in response to the initial stretching sensation, you need to command yourself by saying "let go" or "relax" or "be floppy" or whatever words bring you the relaxing result. The other parts of this stretching method are so effective that this part, the command to relax, only makes the

13

rest easier and initially less uncomfortable.

Sensation: As long as you are alive and active, you will always feel the sensations in your muscles when you are stretching them. This is because even when you are standing still, the muscles on the front and the back of your body are acting in concert to keep you from falling over. That is, most of your muscles spend much of their day contracting, since that is their job. Even after days of bed rest, you feel stiff when you get up to walk around because your muscles have been in various states of contraction. If you don't feel the stretching sensation when you are doing stretches, either you are not putting your body in the correct positions or you have completed the process.

People come in many different packages. Tight-ligamented people easily feel all the stretches in this book. So do "normal"-jointed people. What you should know is that even loose-ligamented people feel these stretches in their muscles each time they do them if they do them correctly. Feeling the sensation of stretching your muscles is just as important as breathing. You must feel the stretch! Then you can accomplish the "melt," the wonderful sensation of relaxed, stretched muscles.

Be Strong and Know Why

The word *strength* means different things to different people. To some, it means being able to lift heavy weights; to others, it means being able to run a marathon in record time or having large, "well-developed" muscles. People's use of the word often indicates what kind of strength they want. Muscles can be large but not have the power to move quickly; and they can be strong and powerful and not be large. Muscles can also be powerful but not have endurance. Having an adequate amount of strength, endurance, and power is most desirable for most people. For each of these goals, there is a specific way of training. You can build strength and endurance at the same time by using the kind of isotonic strengthening exercises in this book. Then you will have muscles that have the power to do what you want to do.

In their book *Total Fitness in 30 Minutes a Week* (New York:

Simon and Schuster, 1975), Laurence E. Morehouse and Leonard Gross state that strength has three aspects: basic strength, endurance, and power. Strength is task specific, which means you need to practice what you want to do in order to do it with power, precision, and control.

There are two popular ways that people use to build strength, which very simply means the ability to do the work by holding and manipulating weight. In power lifting, you lift a heavy weight, hold it, and put it down one or two times. That kind of strength building creates bulky muscles and gives you static strength. The other way to increase strength is called isokinetic, a version of isotonic. In this kind of strength building, you lift small amounts of weight slowly, up and down (against gravity) with equal resistance and speed for many repetitions, until you are very tired, then you repeat the lifting once more for the overload effect. Muscle biopsies of people who have built strength both ways show that both build similar amounts of strength, but muscles from power lifting do not have as much aerobic capacity. That is, they don't have as many spaces in their cell tissue that allow free passage of oxygen. The power-lifting type of strength building, therefore, builds muscles that have very little endurance capacity.

You should understand that different ways of strengthening your muscles bring you different results. If you are clear about why you are getting stronger, then you will know how to go about achieving your goal. The strengthening exercises in this book are isotonic because isotonic exercises build basic strength, and the instructions are written so that they are really isokinetic. This means that your muscles experience equal and uniform resistance from the weight of your body parts going up against gravity and coming down resisting gravity's pull. For the most part, you need no other weights than the ones built into your body.

To summarize: You need to provide your muscles with adequate stretching and to balance this with strengthening exercises that build strong muscles with good endurance capacity. Then you can do any activity you choose to do. By doing your chosen activity with your muscles ready to respond to your commands, you will continue to increase your power to do that activity and enjoy your improvement.

3 Keys to Using This Book

Below you will find lists of the exercises to use for:

- All Active People
- Beginners
- Rush Days — the Irreducible Minimum
- Dancers and Professional Athletes
- Emphasis on Legs
- Emphasis on Upper Body
- People Who Stand a Lot
- Sedentary People
- Inactive People (Confined to Bed or a Chair)
- Counteracting Tension
- Back Care

Turn to the list that matches your needs and do the exercises in the order in which they are listed. Each exercise has its own number which is also on the top corner of the page where it is found in the book. Before you turn to the lists, read the following guidelines to get a better understanding of how the lists are arranged and how to use them.

When you first start your exercise program, be sure to read the anatomical description for each part of your body that you are exercising. Each chapter starts with a brief, nontechnical description of the bones, joints, and muscles in that particular area, which should help you understand why the exercises are designed the way they are.

Warm-up

Experts agree that you should warm up before exercising, but few agree on how long you should warm up or what you should do. Basically, it's agreed you should do something to raise your core temperature above its resting state. That means you should not just fall out of bed and start to exercise but should wait at least 20 minutes after you get up from sleeping or resting before you exercise. Many explanations say that as you warm up you should start to sweat a little, but that will depend on how easily and how long it takes you to start to sweat.

What you can do to warm up varies a lot. You can run in place and wiggle all over for 30 seconds to a minute. You can push against a wall for a minute. You can walk around the room briskly for 3 to 5 minutes. If you land carefully, with your heels coming down to the ground and your knees bending, you can do jumping jacks for a minute. These warm-ups are necessary if you have been sedentary or resting before your exercise session. If you have rushed from work to the gym at lunchtime or hurried to an aerobic dance class after work, you have done more than your share of warming up, technically.

But warming up should mean more than *just* starting to sweat or raising your core temperature. It is hard to put into words, but you should feel something in your body, particularly in your muscles. The term used here for this experience is *readying*. Readying exercises are designed to stretch the muscles you are going to contract or strengthen and to strengthen the muscles you are likely to stretch during your activity or exercise, be it dancing, typing, running, weight lifting, or playing the piano. Do the kind of warm-up that seems most appropriate to your needs, your body, and your activity.

Some instructions say not to stretch before you warm up. This warning probably refers to the percussive or bouncing type of stretching or stretches done in dangerous positions. There are no dangerous stretches or stretching positions in this book, so you need not worry about that problem. If you do the stretching exercises according to the directions, you should experience little or no soreness and take no risks with your body. It is, however, important not to overdo a good thing, so stretch only as long as you feel the relaxing sensation in your muscles, then stop.

Exercise Guidelines

You learned in Chapter 2, "Principles of Stretching and Strengthening," that your muscles only contract on their own; they don't stretch on their own. And you learned that balancing stretching with strengthening keeps your muscles in optimal condition so you can use them for whatever purpose you want. Now you will learn about the order in which to do these readying exercises so that you will get the most benefit with the least discomfort.

1. *Ready before and equalize after.* Before and after your activity, you need to stretch the muscles that you will contract the most during the activity. For instance, when you walk, run, or jog, you will contract and strengthen your leg and buttocks muscle, so you need to stretch these before and after walking, running, or jogging.

Why is it so important to stretch afterward? Remember that muscle tissue is like gelatin. It melts when it is warm and hardens when it cools. If you sit down for a while after you run, an hour later when you want to get up your body is very hard to move. That is because your muscles hardened, cooled down, in their contracted state. If you stretch your leg and buttocks muscles after you run, an hour later you will have little or no residual tightness in your muscles.

A rule of thumb when following the lists in this chapter: Do the stretches and strengthening exercises before your workout and repeat all the stretches afterward.

2. *The order counts.* The lists of exercises that follow are in the order that you should do them. For instance, if possible, always do shoulder stretches before neck stretches and strengthening exercises. That is because your shoulder mus-

cles are the topmost layer of muscle around your neck. When you stretch these first, you will experience less tightness in your neck muscles than if you had stretched your neck muscles first.

If you do strengthening exercises for your shoulders before you stretch them, they will relax more easily when you stretch them properly, because when you strengthen your muscles, you also tire them. When your muscles are tired, they will stretch more easily.

The order in which you stretch your leg muscles is important but varies according to your body and your activity. You will have to experiment with the following pairs of stretches. Before you stretch your hamstrings, always stretch your calf muscles. And before you do a Pretzel or Half Pretzel (exercises 56, 57), always do any of the quadricep stretches in Chapter 11. But you can start with the pair quadriceps/Pretzel and then do the calf/hamstring pair or you can start with calf/hamstring and then do quadriceps/Pretzel.

If you do Ankle Crisscross and Sand Scraping (exercises 91, 92) before you do your calf stretches, you will feel less tightness and achieve more stretch in your calf. On the other hand, you may want to save the ankle and foot readying exercises until just before you set out to run or dance or jump because your feet will be the most ready to lift and receive your body weight. Your specific needs will sometimes determine the order of your exercises. The lists are arranged in the best possible order for most people and most activities.

3. *The harder you work the more you need to get your muscles ready.* Professional athletes and dancers spend a lot of time getting ready for their activities. The closer you push yourself to your limit, the more your muscles will need to be ready to meet that challenge. When you push yourself, you also push your body's unevennesses, old sprains, strains, and injuries. The more time you take to get your body ready, the more you will enjoy your activity without risk. For instance, there is the Standing Hamstring Stretch (exercise 71) and the Triple Hamstring Stretch (exercise 72). Dancers need to do both. If you are a runner competing in a race, you should also do both stretches because your legs will be very ready to go, readier than if you did just one of them.

4. *Specific needs require special care.* If you are recovering from an injury, you need to take more time to ready the injured area (see Chapter 16). If you have been inactive for a while, you need to start out slowly and be patient. Your former muscle capacity will return if you work carefully. If you have very tight joints and your muscles are extra tight, then you will need to take more time to stretch than the suggested 30 seconds to a minute. Take 1 to 2 minutes for each stretch position. You will see wonderful results, but it will take extra time to get them. If your ligaments are very loose, then you, too, will need to adjust your body to the stretch positions and take longer to ready your body for activity. Throughout the book, there are guidelines for how you loose-ligamented people can adjust your bodies to feel the stretches.

Exercise Lists

ALL ACTIVE PEOPLE

40–45 minutes for the whole set

If your work or sport uses your whole body actively, then you can use this set of exercises. Use the entire series before and the stretches only after. Take time to do the entire series on the days you do not work or play. This series balances stretching with strengthening, except for strengthening your thighs because your total body activity probably gives you enough thigh strengthening.

36, 37. Finger Circles and Finger Presses. Do at some time during the day.
15. Chicken, or **14.** Hug the World
39. Cone-shaped Stretch
26. Push-ups of some form, or **25, 28, 29**
18. Hanging from a Bar
10. Shoulder Stretch from Below
11. Shoulder Stretch from the Side with **21.** Wrist Stretch
20. Triceps Stretch
12. Shoulder Stretch from Above
1, 2, 3. Neck Stretches: Center, Side, Diagonal
6. Rotating Neck Stretch

4, 5, 7. Head Raises: Center, Diagonal, Side and Rotating

58. Hip Curl

47. Curl-downs or some form of abdominal strengthening: **45, 46, 48**

61. Sitting Quadriceps Stretch and **62.** Salt Shaker

55. Half Pretzel, or **56.** Pretzel

85. Standing Calf Stretch

87. A-frame Calf Stretch

66. Deep Lunge

71. Standing Hamstring Stretch

76. Three-Part Inner Thigh Stretch

95. Inchworm

91. Ankle Crisscross

92. Sand Scraping

89. One-Footed Heel Raises, or **90.** Slow Motion Jumping and then **85, 87**

BEGINNERS

40–45 minutes for the whole set

These exercises can help you start to build a balance of stretch and strength in your body. When these no longer challenge you, move on to the list for All Active People.

48 **13.** Snow Angel

85 **39.** Cone-shaped Stretch

68-69 **28, 29.** Front and Side Wall Push-ups

43 **10.** Shoulder Stretch from Below   *60*

45 **11.** Shoulder Stretch from the Side with **21.** Wrist Stretch

46 **12.** Shoulder Stretch from Above

1, 2, 3. Neck Stretches: Center, Side, Diagonal   *32 33 34*

4, 5. Head Raises: Center and Diagonal   *34 35*

6. Rotating Neck Stretch   *36*

94 **45.** Pussy Cat

95 **46.** Leg-Arm-Head Lifts   *126*

124 **61.** Sitting Quadriceps Stretch and **62.** Salt Shaker

114 **55.** Half Pretzel

167- **85.** Standing Calf Stretch

136- **71.** Standing Hamstring Stretch

141 **73.** Backward Leg Circles   *167*

133 **68.** Leg Extensions and then **85.** Standing Calf Stretch

180 **95.** Inchworm

RUSH DAYS — IRREDUCIBLE MINIMUM

If your day is so busy that you will only have a few minutes to do any stretching and strengthening, do the following exercises:

85. Standing Calf Stretch
71. Standing Hamstring Stretch
47. Curl-downs of some form, or **45, 46, 48**
11. Shoulder Stretch from the Side with **21.** Wrist Stretch
1. Center Neck Stretch
39. Cone-shaped Stretch
50. Door Frame Pull

DANCERS AND PROFESSIONAL ATHLETES

If you push your body to its limit and challenge yourself to achieve new skills, you need this very full series of readying exercises. When you complete the series, you should feel very ready to perform.

15. Chicken, or **14.** Hug the World
41. Back Rib Stretch
61. Sitting Quadriceps Stretch with **11.** Shoulder Stretch from the Side
56. Pretzel with **10.** Shoulder Stretch from Below
12. Shoulder Stretch from Above
1, 2, 3. Neck Stretches: Center, Side, Diagonal
4, 5. Head Raises: Center and Diagonal
58. Hip Curl with **83.** Leg Extensions
47. Curl-downs
84. Sitting Calf Stretch, or **88.** Phone Book Calf Stretch
85. Standing Calf Stretch
87. A-frame Calf Stretch with **27.** A-frame Push-ups

66. Deep Lunge
71. Standing Hamstring Stretch
72. Triple Hamstring Stretch
75. Inner and Outer Thigh Lifts
54. Open Tailor Sit
76. Three-Part Inner Thigh Stretch
78. Outer Thigh Lifts, Sitting
79. Three-Part Straddle Stretch
81. Strengthening from Straddle Stretch
55. Half Pretzel, or **56.** Pretzel
95. Inchworm
97. Hiccup
91. Ankle Crisscross
92. Sand Scraping
30. Seagulls
31. Cormorants
32. Mallards

EMPHASIS ON LEGS

If your work or sport emphasizes your legs, as in running or aerobic dance, you need to follow the list for All Active People and then make sure you balance stretch and strength in your upper body with the strength and flexibility of your lower body. So to that list after Push-ups, you should add:

24. Cutting Cheese (on the floor with small weights)

EMPHASIS ON UPPER BODY

If your activities challenge your upper body, as in weight lifting or drumming, you need to stretch your upper body adequately and make sure that your legs have a balance of stretching and strengthening.

39. Cone-shaped Stretch
10. Shoulder Stretch from Below
11. Shoulder Stretch from the Side with **21.** Wrist Stretch
20. Triceps Stretch
12. Shoulder Stretch from Above

1, 2, 3. Neck Stretches: Center, Side, Diagonal
6. Rotating Neck Stretch
4, 5, 7. Head Raises: Center, Diagonal, Side and Rotating
47. Curl-downs, or **49.** Wall Curl-downs
50. Door Frame Pull
51. Super Back Rest, or **52.** Paul Williams's Back Stretch
61. Sitting Quadriceps Stretch and **62.** Salt Shaker
54. Open Tailor Sit
55. Half Pretzel, or **56.** Pretzel
85. Standing Calf Stretch
87. A-frame Calf Stretch
66. Deep Lunge
71. Standing Hamstring Stretch
76. Three-Part Inner Thigh Stretch
95. Inchworm
91. Ankle Crisscross
92. Sand Scraping
89. One-Footed Heel Raises, or **90.** Slow Motion Jumping
and then **85** and **87**

PEOPLE WHO STAND A LOT

You can do these exercises while you are standing. (Only one requires that you sit down.) You can also do any of them at any time. They will relieve your muscles from the strain of standing.

28, 29. Wall Push-ups, Front and Side
39. Cone-shaped Stretch
18. Hanging from a Bar, or chin-ups
10. Shoulder Stretch from Below
11. Shoulder Stretch from the Side with **21.** Wrist Stretch
20. Triceps Stretch
12. Shoulder Stretch from Above
1, 2, 3. Neck Stretches: Center, Side, Diagonal
44. Isometric Abdominal Strengthening
63. Standing Quadriceps Stretch
66. Deep Lunge
77. Outer Thigh Lifts (standing)
85. Standing Calf Stretch

71. Standing Hamstring Stretch
55. Half Pretzel or **56.** Pretzel
95. Inchworm
91. Ankle Crisscross
92. Sand Scraping
89. One-Footed Heel Raises, or **90.** Slow Motion Jumping

SEDENTARY PEOPLE

If you ride to work and sit at your job, then much of your day is spent in a sedentary manner. If you have not yet found time for any regular exercise, you need these readying exercises and some kind of aerobic activity to build the cardiovascular capacity of your heart and lungs. You need to do some kind of vigorous physical activity at least three times a week. Make sure to choose something you really enjoy doing.

The list for Beginners or All Active People may best fit your needs if you are ready for that level of stretching and strengthening. Pay special attention to the abdominal strengthening exercises and alignment guidelines.

INACTIVE PEOPLE: CONFINED TO BED

If you are confined to your bed or a chair for any length of time, your body will begin to cry out for some form of muscle use. Check with your doctor and physical therapist before you start any exercise program; then try this list, carefully.

13. Snow Angel
16. Shoulder Shrugs
6. Rotating Neck Stretch
4, 5. Head Raises: Center and Diagonal
7. Side and Rotating Head Raises
33–38. All the hand and wrist exercises
57. Kegel Exercise
58. Hip Curl
44. Isometric Abdominal Strengthening

46. Leg-Arm-Head Lifts
51. Super Back Rest
52. Paul Williams's Back Stretch
53. Chiropractic Position
72. Triple Hamstring Stretch (lying part only)
68. Leg Extensions (on your back)
64. Side Lying Quadriceps Stretch
77. Outer Thigh Lifts, Lying
91. Ankle Crisscross
93. Toe Curls and Uncurls
94. Toe Open and Close
Breathing (Chapter 15)

INACTIVE PEOPLE: CONFINED TO A CHAIR

39. Cone-shaped Stretch
23. Arm Circles
24. Cutting Cheese
14. Hug the World
10. Shoulder Stretch from Below
12. Shoulder Stretch from Above
16. Shoulder Shrugs
17. Shoulder Circles
19. Lifting from Your Chair
1, 2, 3. Neck Stretches: Center, Side, Diagonal
21. Wrist Stretch
22. Forearm Stretch
33–38. All the hand and wrist exercises
44. Isometric Abdominal Strengthening
57. Kegel Exercise
59. Jumping in Your Chair
68. Leg Extensions (sitting)
72. Triple Hamstring Stretch (sitting part only)
91. Ankle Crisscross
92. Sand Scraping
93. Toe Curls and Uncurls
94. Toe Open and Close
95. Inchworm

COUNTERACTING TENSION

If you feel daily tension and stress settle in your muscles, try these exercises. They will relieve at least the physical side of your tension, because they have chosen to counteract tension in the places in your body that are likely to carry tension. You can do any of these at any time.

Breathing (Chapter 15)
13. Snow Angel
39. Cone-shaped Stretch
10. Shoulder Stretch from Below
11. Shoulder Stretch from the Side with **21.** Wrist Stretch
12. Shoulder Stretch from Above
1, 2, 3, 6. Neck Stretches: Center, Side, Diagonal, Rotating
4, 5. Head Raises: Center and Diagonal
50. Door Frame Pull
51. Super Back Rest
58. Hip Curl
54. Open Tailor Sit
88. Phone Book Calf Stretch
91. Ankle Crisscross

BACK CARE

Your back is very vulnerable. How you sit, stand, walk, work, play, and even sleep can make your back comfortable or uncomfortable. The following exercises are particularly helpful for maintaining your back in the best possible state. See Chapter 16 for many more guidelines in caring for your back.

50. Door Frame Pull
13. Snow Angel
10, 11, 12. Shoulder Stretches: from Below, Side, Above
1, 2, 3. Neck Stretches: Center, Side, Diagonal
6. Rotating Neck Stretch
4, 5, 7. Head Raises: Center, Diagonal, Side and Rotating
58. Hip Curl
45. Pussy Cat and **46.** Leg-Arm-Head Lifts
51. Super Back Rest, or **52.** Paul Williams's Back Stretch

53. Chiropractic Position
64. Side Lying Quadriceps Stretch
54. Open Tailor Sit
55. Half Pretzel, or **56.** Pretzel
85. Standing Calf Stretch, or **88.** Phone Book Calf Stretch
87. A-frame Calf Stretch
72. Triple Hamstring Stretch

*

As you follow these lists of exercises, you will be reading around in many different chapters. Read the introductory words for the exercises near the ones you are doing to see if they will fit your needs, then try them. Be sure to read the anatomical descriptions of each part of the body that you are exercising to understand why the exercises are designed as they are. Refer to Chapter 16 if you have any sore areas in your body that need special care. When you follow these guidelines and do the exercises, you will be able to keep your muscles moving and keep your body in motion.

4 Your Neck

Anatomy

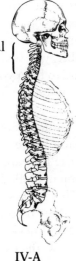

cervical
spine

IV-A

The skull and the seven vertebrae of the neck (cervical) portion of the spine are the major bones in this area of the body *(IV-A)*. The skull is very firmly attached to the topmost vertebra, called the atlas. The joint between the skull and atlas lets you nod your head forward and back. The skull and atlas sit on top of the next vertebra, the axis, and it is the joint between them that lets you rotate your head. Unlike the atlas and the axis, which have different shapes, the other five neck vertebrae all have a similar shape, which enables you to move your neck fully: forward, up to vertical, back, to each side, ear to shoulder, and in rotation. You can move your head by itself as well as with your neck. These bones are connected by very strong ligaments.

You can move your bones because of muscle actions. The job of the muscles of the neck and head is twofold. They hold your head up above your upright body so you can use all your senses, which are located in your skull. That is their static, holding, balancing job. And they allow you to move your head, along with your neck, to do the actions that go along with the use of your senses when you see, smell, and listen; and they enable you to talk, eat, drink, and so forth.

You have groups of muscles on all sides of your joints that

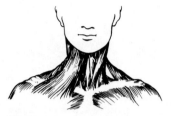

IV-B
front neck muscles

enable you to move in the ways these joints allow. So, the muscles just for your head move it forward, back, and in rotation. The neck muscles on the back of your neck move your head and neck up from a forward position or back from a vertical position to look at the sky. Those same muscles help move your head and neck sideways and in rotation. Muscles in front of your spine help keep your neck and head vertical. And the muscles in front of your neck bend your neck and head forward and move your head sideways and in rotation. Under your chin are muscles that help you swallow *(IV-B)*.

Unless you are lying down, your neck muscles are on constant duty to keep your 10- to 12-pound head upright. That is no easy task, for two reasons. First, you need to move your head in many ways during your daily activities. Second, the center of gravity of your head is in front of the joint where your skull sits on your atlas, so the weight of your head is always pulling forward. The action of your muscles is to keep it vertical, so the muscles on the back of your neck are kept busy pulling your head back up. This is a major reason for any tightness you may feel in the back of your neck.

Throughout this book, the instructions remind you to bring your chin in. If you make this a habit, you will be using the neck muscles in front of your spine to help you keep your head "on straight" and maintain a more comfortable head alignment.

Here is one other interesting bit of information about neck muscles: the muscles that control the side movements of your neck differ from those that control the forward movement (called flexion) and backward movement (called extension, and sometimes hyperextension). The flexors, which move your head and neck forward, have their own names, and the extensors, which move your head and neck back or up, have other names. When the flexors work, the extensors relax or stretch, and vice versa. When you move your head and neck to the side, the muscles that control this action cooperate with each other. One side contracts, or shortens, and the other does a lengthening contraction, called an eccentric contraction. Remember, the job of the neck muscles is to keep your head upright, so the muscles on either side of your neck co-contract to do their job. The muscles that control the lateral movement of your neck have the same names and are attached in the same place on both sides of your neck. These muscles cause your head to flip back up automatically when you start to fall asleep sitting in class or on a bus and your head falls sideways. (This is also why traditional neck circles do not relax tight neck muscles. To relax muscles, you need to stretch them, and neck circles mainly contract them.)

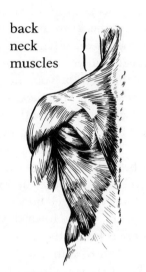

back
neck
muscles

IV-C

The tightest muscles in your neck are in the back *(IV-C)*. They become extra tight from not keeping your head "on straight" in many daily activities, such as eating, driving, reading, even just sitting slumped. These muscles need stretching. You can reduce the discomfort of a tension head-ache by doing the neck stretches in this chapter. The weak-est muscles are in the front of your neck, because when your head is not vertically aligned, you are not only contracting the back muscles, you are also stretching the ones in front. They need strengthening. A "forward head" position can cause pain underneath your shoulder blades, so proper head alignment and a balance of stretching and strengthening ex-ercises can eliminate this problem. Chapter 16 has guide-lines for taking care of a sore back, as well as other problems related to head alignment, such as a sore neck, a crick in the neck, and sore shoulders.

Exercises

Before you do these neck exercises, always do the three shoulder stretches (exercises 10–12).

READYING POSITION: During the entire time you are doing these exercises, remember to keep your jaw relaxed and your head "on straight." That means keep it in proper alignment. What is proper head alignment? Feel that the top back of your head, the place where your spine goes up into your skull, is being pulled up. Then your ears will be over your shoulders and your head will be in its proper place. You don't want your head forward, down, or tipped back. These nonvertical positions use your neck and shoulder muscles unevenly. Whenever you do these exercises for your neck —

and all the others in this book — remember to align your head correctly and relax your jaw.

1

CENTER NECK STRETCH

STARTING POSITION: Extend your neck up in a long vertical line. The reason to stretch your neck up as much as possible is that in everyday life your head often slips forward and down. Then your seven cervical vertebrae are unstacked and the normal curve in the back of your neck is exaggerated. Relax your face muscles and your jaw. Open your mouth slightly so you won't clench your teeth. Now move your chin in toward your neck as though someone were about to push you in the face. Keep your chin close to your neck while you do this stretch, but don't feel as though you are going to choke. This position lets you use the inner neck muscles to balance your skull on your neck bones.

THE STRETCH: (1) Curve your head down toward your chest as you were trying to see something at the bottom of your chin. Keep your chin from touching your chest. This will keep your vertebrae stacked and let you stretch those tight muscles. Place one hand on the back part of the top of your head and gently and continuously pull your head down, *1*. The shape of the stretch is like an upside-down *J*. Feel the stretch pull all along the muscles of the back of your neck, especially up into the lower part of the back of your head. Hold this position for 30 seconds to a minute. {**Troubleshooting:** If you don't feel the stretch sensation in your skull, only below your neck, you may have let your chin move down and your neck move forward. Don't let your chin touch your chest.} (2) In this forward position, turn your head a little to the right, as if starting to shake your head "no," and hold this position for 30 seconds. Now turn your head a little to your left to shake the other half of your "no." Remember to relax your jaw. The pull of your hand should be gentle but not so gentle that you feel no stretch. Repeat Step 1. After completing neck stretches to the side and to the diagonal (exercises 2 and 3), do this Center Neck Stretch

1

again. Then you will feel much less tightness than you did after completing this stretch for the first time.

(See the last paragraph of exercise 3.)

2

SIDE NECK STRETCH

STARTING POSITION: Align your head vertically just as you did for Center Neck Stretch (exercise 1).

THE STRETCH: **(1)** Curve your head sideways to your right so that your ear is over your shoulder. Keep your gaze and your face looking forward, not down or up. Place your right hand on the left top side of your head and gently pull your head toward your right shoulder, *2a*. Hold this position for 30 seconds. **(2)** Relax both shoulders, especially the right, and deliberately keep them down, *2b*. Hold this position for 30 seconds. **(3)** Reach down to the floor with your left arm, *2c*. By doing this you will feel the stretch even more in the neck muscles on your left side. Slowly reach a little forward with your left arm and then reach a little backward while still pulling your arm down. Add 10 to 20 seconds to your total stretch with your arm reaching down. {**Troubleshooting:** Keep your chin in toward your neck, your mouth open, and your jaw relaxed.}

Repeat this stretch to the left, using your left hand to weight your head to the left side.

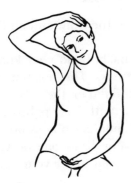

2a

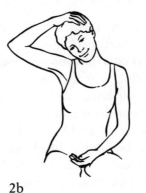

2b

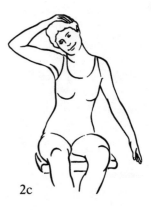

2c

3

DIAGONAL NECK STRETCH

STARTING POSITION: Align your head vertically as you did for the Center Neck Stretch (exercise 1). Place your right hand on the back part of the top of your head. Curve your head forward into the upside-down *J* position. Now put your head and neck on a diagonal by moving them toward your right knee. Next, rotate your head to the left in a small half "no," as in exercise 1. This rotation is a small head tilt and will shift your gaze more toward center front.

THE STRETCH: **(1)** With your right hand on the left back top part of your head, gently pull your head in an upside-down *J* curve, *3*. Hold this stretch for 30 seconds. **(2)** Reach your left arm behind you and pull it down toward the floor in a back diagonal and hold this position for 30 more seconds. You will feel this stretch in the area of your neck where the back and side converge. Repeat the Diagonal Neck Stretch on your left side.

Repeat the Center Neck Stretch (exercise 1). You should now feel less tightness in those muscles. If you round your upper back by pushing back your rib cage, you can feel this stretch below your neck along the muscles on both sides of your spine going down between your shoulder blades. After you do the neck strengthening exercises, the tightness in these muscles will be gone, or at least almost gone.

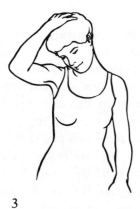

3

4

HEAD RAISES TO THE CENTER

Head raises strengthen the muscles in the front and on the sides of your neck.

STARTING POSITION: Lie on your back. Bend your knees and bring your feet close to your buttocks. This position allows your lower back to be relaxed and flat on the floor. Extend your arms sideways on the floor with your palms up. Relax your shoulders and pull your shoulder blades down. Before beginning head raises, lift your head one or two inches and stretch your neck longer, then lower your head to the floor. Relax your jaw.

THE STRENGTHENING EXERCISE: **(1)** Slowly lift your

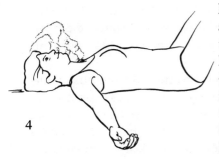

4

head by tucking in your chin and curving your forehead up as though you were trying to see something on the floor between your knees, *4*. Take 4 counts to do this. Keep your head slowly and continuously moving in a curved path. {**Troubleshooting:** Don't stop moving and don't face the ceiling with your neck parallel to the floor. Keep your chin tucked in} **(2)** Reverse this action slowly, as if you were pressing each neck vertebra down to the floor separately. Put your head, with your chin tucked in, down on the floor last. Take 4 slow counts to do this.

5   HEAD RAISES TO THE DIAGONAL

STARTING POSITION: Assume the same starting position as for head raises to the center (exercise 4). Now turn your head (which is resting on the floor) to the right as though you were going to look over your right shoulder, *5a*. Don't bring your head closer to your shoulder by rolling it sideways on the floor. Just rotate it and keep your neck extended straight.

THE STRENGTHENING EXERCISE: **(1)** Lift your head, forehead first, *5b*, in a curved path to look at the floor underneath your right armpit, *5c*. Take 4 counts to do this. It is all right if your left shoulder comes off the floor. **(2)** Now put each vertebra of your neck back down on the floor, with your head last. Take 4 slow counts to do this. Keep your head continuously moving during this up-and-down movement.

Turn your head up to the ceiling and then look over your left shoulder and repeat steps 1 and 2 to your left.

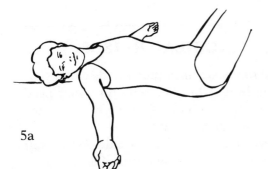

5a

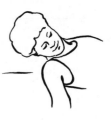

5b   5c

Now repeat Head Raises to the Center and to each side two more times for a total of three sets. {**Troubleshooting:** Be sure to place your neck down on the floor first, not your head.}

To sit up, roll your entire body to the side and push yourself up with your hands. Do the neck stretches (exercises 1–3) again. The little bit of tightness in your neck muscles that remained after you finished the neck stretches earlier should be almost or entirely gone after these neck strengthening exercises. If it is not, try the next set and then repeat the neck stretches.

6   ROTATING NECK STRETCH

This stretch will ready your neck for the Side and Rotating Head Raises (exercise 7).

STARTING POSITION: Lie on your back. Bend your knees and bring your feet close to your buttocks. Extend your arms sideways on the floor with your palms up. Relax your neck to decrease the space between your neck and the floor.

THE STRETCH: Rotate your head to the right as far as is comfortable by trying to look over your right shoulder. Place your right hand on your left cheek and gently press the side of your face farther toward the floor. Hold this position for 30 seconds to a minute. To repeat on the other side, first rotate your head back to the starting position. Keep your chin in. Repeat this stretch to the left.

7   SIDE AND ROTATING HEAD RAISES

If the following head raises are uncomfortable because your neck is stiff and even hurts when you only turn your head from side to side, continue to do the Rotating Neck Stretch (exercise 6) until your neck is less stiff.

STARTING POSITION: Lie on your right side. Bend your right leg to help you keep your body on its side. Use your left hand on the floor in front of your chest to maintain your balance in this side position. Extend your right arm on the floor. Face forward. *7a.*

THE STRENGTHENING EXERCISE: **(1)** Slowly lift your head from the resting position to a vertical position. Your ear is moving toward your left shoulder, *7b,c,d.* Take 4 counts to do this. **(2)** Slowly lower your head back to a horizontal position, but *don't* rest it on your arm, *7e.* You are holding it about 2 inches off the floor. **(3)** Slowly turn your head so you bring your face toward the ceiling, *7f,g,h.* Keep your jaw relaxed and your chin in toward your neck. Take 4 counts to do this. **(4)** Return your head to face forward in 4 counts, *7i.* **(5)** Turn your head so your face looks down at the floor, *7j,k,* taking 4 slow counts. **(6)** Return your head so your face is forward, *7i,* taking 4 slow counts. Repeat these six steps two more times. Rest your head down on your bent arm for a few counts.

Roll over on your left side and repeat the sequence.

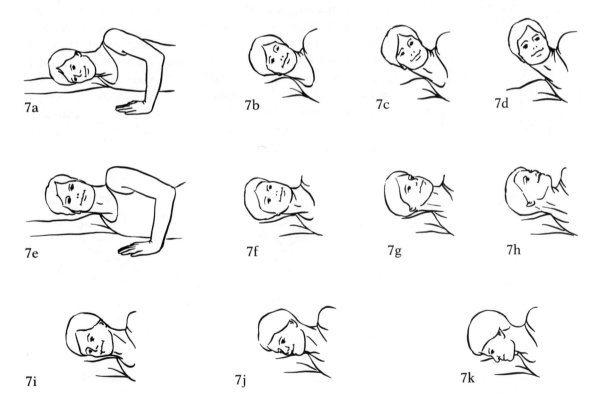

7a   7b   7c   7d

7e   7f   7g   7h

7i   7j   7k

8

CORRECTED HEAD CIRCLES

8a

To protect the disks in your spine, don't do traditional neck circles. Here is a safe way to practice the neck exercises that are part of many warm-up sequences.

STARTING POSITION: Stretch your neck vertically and bring in your chin. Relax your jaw.

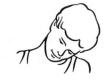

8b

THE COORDINATION EXERCISE: **(1)** Slowly lower your left ear toward your left shoulder as though you were beginning the Side Neck Stretch (exercise 2), *8a.* Take 2 counts to do this. **(2)** Slowly lower your face toward the floor, keeping your chin in and your neck vertebrae as vertical as possible, *8b,c,* taking 2 counts. **(3)** Reach your right ear toward and then above your right shoulder, *8d,e,* taking 2 counts. **(4)** Slowly bring your head up to a vertical position, *8f,* feeling the muscles on the left side of your face contracting and doing the lifting. Take 2 counts to do this. Repeat this sequence starting on the right side. Repeat this side, center, side, and up pathway two more times. Imagine that your head is pushing something heavy while making this path and you will feel your neck muscles control the movement of your head and not the reverse. Your head weighs 10 to 12 pounds, and if you let it fall to the side, forward, to the other side, and up, momentum will carry your head and your muscles will be mildly yanked. You can increase the speed of these circles to match the ticking of the clock and consciously continue to feel your neck muscles controlling the weight of your head.

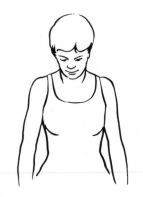

8c

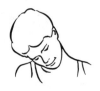

8d

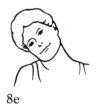

8e

8f

9

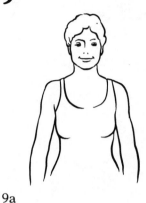

9a

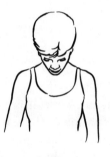

9b

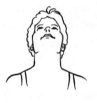

9c

FLOOR AND CEILING

This exercise teaches you to align your head correctly while looking at the floor or watching birds and airplanes in the sky.

STARTING POSITION: With your chin in and your jaw relaxed, extend your neck vertically, *9a.*

THE COORDINATION EXERCISE: (1) Keep your chin in while you slowly press your forehead down and forward, *9b.* Feel the muscles in the back of your neck stretch. Take 2 counts to do this. {**Troubleshooting:** Don't let your chin touch your chest.} **(2)** Lift your head so that your neck is vertical and in the starting position, *9a.* Take 2 counts to do this. **(3)** Lift your face so it is parallel to the ceiling and turn it slightly to one side or the other, *9c.* This way you will keep the tips of your vertebrae from bumping against each other and the movement will be more comfortable. Take 2 counts to do this. {**Troubleshooting:** Try talking while you do this. If you can talk easily, you have done this correctly by lifting your face and rocking your atlas vertebra on its axis joint while keeping your neck vertebrae vertically stacked. If you can't talk, you have partially closed your windpipe by dropping your head back passively. Dropping it can be harmful to your disks.} **(4)** Slowly bring your chin down so your head is vertical again, *9a.* Take 2 counts.

You can increase the speed of Floor and Ceiling to match the ticking of the clock, but keep in mind the image of pushing something heavy with your head. This way you will continue to feel your neck muscles working and you will not allow momentum to control the weight of your head.

5 Your Shoulders

Anatomy

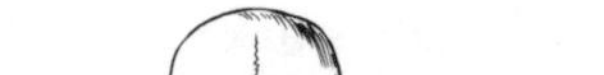

The structure of your shoulder is unusual. First, it is multi-jointed. The shoulder girdle is a combination of three bones. The shoulder blade, or scapula, is in the back on top of the rib cage and attaches above the arm bone to the collarbone, or clavicle *(V-A)*. The other end of the clavicle is in front and attaches under the chin to the breastbone, or sternum *(V-B)*. The third bone is the upper arm bone, or humerus, which attaches to a shallow socket on the top corner of the scapula *(V-C)*. The oddest part of this structure is that the edge of the scapula near the spine is free-floating, for it is held in place with muscles, not ligaments. The other bones are held together with strong ligaments.

When you move your entire arm your shoulder blade moves, and when you move your shoulder blade your arm moves; the movement of these bones is cooperative. Your shoulder blade moves up and down, outward around your rib cage (called outward rotation), and back to place, down and around (called inward rotation). The range of motion in your arm is very great because of the relatively loose style of bone attachment. Your arm at your shoulder moves around in a full circle at a right angle to your body, as well as around in a side to side circle in front of your body, like

shoulder:
back view

V-A

lower back
and hips
with femur

shoulder:
front view

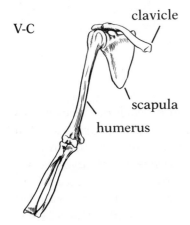

V-B

the hand of a clock. You can make this kind of a circle behind you as well, but the range is much more limited. You can also rotate your entire arm inward and outward. This means that when your arm is extended down at your side, you can turn it clockwise so that your palm, elbow, and upper arm are facing out, away from your body; and you can turn it counterclockwise, facing in.

The muscle structure of the shoulder girdle enables you to move your bones in these various ways *(V-D, V-E)*. There are muscles to lift and lower your shoulder blade and clavicle, to open and close your shoulder blades together, and to help them rotate outward and inward. There are muscles to lift and lower your arm forward and back, up and down, side to side, and around. Because your arm attaches to your scapula, the muscles that enable you to move your scapula also work when you move your arm.

It is important to know about the relatively loose structure of the shoulder girdle. The term *girdle* refers to all three bones, their joints, and their muscles. The shoulder joint refers to the attachment of the humerus in its shallow socket of the scapula. Because this socket is so shallow, four of the

V-C

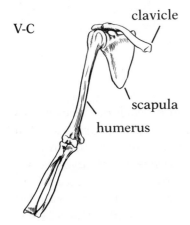

clavicle

scapula

humerus

shoulder and arm:
front view

V-D

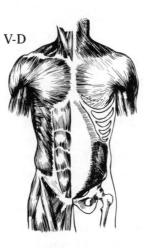

front chest and
shoulder muscles

V-E

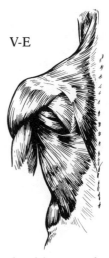

shoulder muscles,
back view

muscles that move the arm are also structured to support and even hold the humerus in its socket. These are the rotator cuff muscles. How well your shoulder works depends on how well balanced your muscles are, that is, on whether they are equally strong and stretched. Because human beings no longer hang from trees as we did when we were evolving from primates, the muscles that hold the shoulder blades down and together are often stretched too much and weak. In fact, studies show that the downward depressors of the shoulder blade are the weakest in the human body. The result of this imbalance is that the bones of the shoulder girdle do not readily stay in their proper positions, which means that your muscles and ligaments do not always support your arm adequately or correctly when you move it.

The exercises in this chapter emphasize creating this balance of stretch and strength in your shoulder girdle muscles. In particular, they stretch your front shoulder muscles, which are often too tight, and strengthen your downward depressors, the muscles in back that hold your shoulder blades down and together. The exercises are designed to maintain correct placement of your shoulder girdle bones and therefore prevent injury and immobility.

Chapter 16 has guidelines for caring for a sore shoulder.

Exercises

READYING POSITION: When you do each of the exercises in this book, please remember to put your head "on straight." That means: **(1)** lengthen your neck upward; **(2)** keep your chin relaxed and in; and **(3)** feel as though you are hanging by the top of your spine (or from the place where your spine would come out of your skull if it extended straight up from where it holds up your skull). That place is in the back of your skull, straight up the back of your neck.

To ready your shoulders for each of these exercises, pull your shoulder blades down. When you let the muscles of your shoulder blades relax, whether you are sitting or standing, the tight muscles in the front of your shoulders are likely to pull your upper body into a "round shoulder" posture. If you do any exercise in this "round shoulder" position, you may hurt your shoulder joint. And the result of these stretches and strengthening exercises will not be as beneficial.

It is not easy to keep your shoulder blades pulled down. Before you do the exercises in this chapter, do Shoulder Shrugs (exercise 16) so you can practice pulling down your shoulder blades.

After you do the stretches for the front of your shoulder muscles and then do the strengthening exercises that specifically tone the downward depressors of your shoulder blades, you will be able to keep your shoulders more easily in their proper position and prevent the "round shoulder" position. If you also keep your head aligned, you'll be better able to keep your shoulder blades in place. This correct posture will, in turn, give your lungs more room to expand and relax freely, and then you may fatigue less easily because you will be supplying your body with an even flow of oxygen.

*

To stretch your muscles in the front part of your shoulders, you will use three different positions: **(1)** in back, from below; **(2)** from the side; and **(3)** from above to the back.

10   SHOULDER STRETCH FROM BELOW

STARTING POSITION: You will need a rope, towel, or belt to hold. Sit or stand with your arms hanging down at your sides. Pull your shoulder blades down and make sure to keep them down. Reach your arms behind your back and hold the rope so that your hands are 6 to 10 inches apart. Remember to keep your head aligned and your chin in.

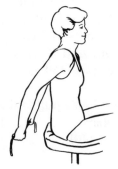

10a

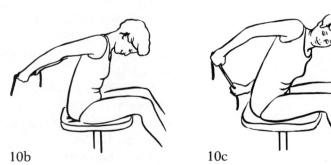

10b   10c

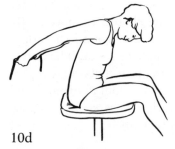

10d

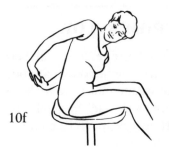

10e

10f

THE STRETCH: Lift up both your arms 4 to 6 inches. Keep your elbows relaxed or a little bent, *10a*. Bend your upper body forward as though starting to bow. This position helps to lift your arms a little higher, *10b*. Now turn your upper body to the right so that your left shoulder is down toward the floor and your right shoulder is up toward the ceiling. Lift your arms up more than they were in the starting-to-stretch position, *10c*. You should feel the stretch more strongly in the right shoulder in this turned position. You can feel this stretch in the front of your shoulder, between your shoulder blades (what you feel here is a contraction), and on the side of your chest under and behind your armpits. Hold this turned position for 30 seconds to a minute. Then turn your upper body so that you tip your right shoulder down to the floor. Now, with your left shoulder up, you'll feel the stretching in front of and behind that shoulder. Hold that position for 30 seconds to a minute. The position for the next step is the first position, with your upper body bent forward and both hands holding the rope. Now lift your arms so that you feel the stretch in the front of both your shoulders. You should be able to lift your arms higher now than you were able to when you began this stretch, *10d*. Hold your arms up for 30 seconds to a minute. Be sure to keep your shoulder blades down and your elbows bent.

You are now going to repeat this sequence with your hands clasped together, *10e,f*. If the angle of pull is too great to be comfortable with your hands together, then continue to use the rope and move your hands closer together. Repeat

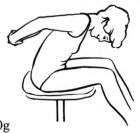

10g

the sequence with your left shoulder up toward the ceiling and your right one down toward the floor. Hold the position 30 seconds to a minute. Then turn your upper body so that your right shoulder is up and your left shoulder is down, *10g*. Hold that position for 30 seconds to a minute. Now return to your first bent-forward position and lift up both of your arms. You should be able to raise your arms higher than at the end of the first stretch sequence.

11   SHOULDER STRETCH FROM THE SIDE

STARTING POSITION: With your left side to the wall, stand an arm's length away from it. Extend your left arm out and put your hand on the wall so that your wrist is flexed and your fingers are back, not up or forward, *11a*. If your wrist is too uncomfortable in this position, place your hand around a door frame so your fingers are bent. Make sure to keep your shoulder blade down and to relax (not lock) your elbow. Keep your head aligned and your chin in.

THE STRETCH: Turn your entire body to the right by moving your feet. You are trying to turn your back to the wall, *11b*. You will not need to turn very far (nor can you) before you feel a strong stretch across the front of your chest and shoulder. You may also feel this stretch in your wrist and forearm. If you want to feel it more, lean toward your left

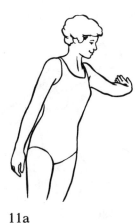

11a

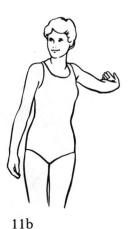

11b

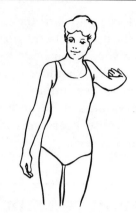

shoulder by transferring your weight forward on your feet, *11c.* Hold this stretch for 30 seconds to a minute.

Repeat this stretch for your right arm by extending it out to the wall or door frame and turning to your left.

If you are like most people, your body is unevenly tight, so you will probably feel this stretch more strongly in the shoulder of the arm with which you write. Hold the stretch longer on your tighter side. Another way to accomplish a similar side arm stretch will be described with the quadriceps stretch (exercise 61) on the floor in Chapter ll.

11c

12   SHOULDER STRETCH FROM ABOVE

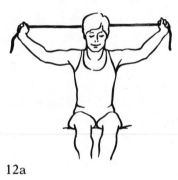

STARTING POSITION: You will need a rope, belt, broomstick, or towel to hold. Sit on the floor, a chair, or a stool. The seated position protects your lower back.

THE STRETCH: Hold the rope with your hands about 3 feet apart. Extend your arms out in front of you. Keep your elbows relaxed. Now lift your arms up and over your head. Carefully move them back to the place where you feel tightness in the top front of your shoulder joint. At that place, stop moving your arms back, *12a.* Instead, move both of your arms and the rope to the right. Just move your arms; don't tilt your body. You have moved the triangle of your arms and the rope sideways about 6 to 8 inches in order to stretch one shoulder at a time. Bend your right elbow and use your right hand to pull the left extended arm back to

12a

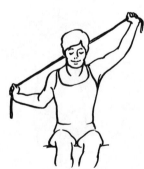

12b

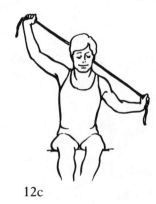

12c

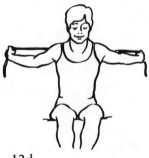

12d

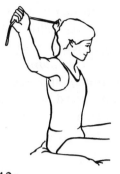

12e

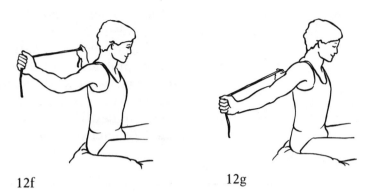

12f

12g

stretch the tight place you felt when you started this stretch. Position the pulling hand below and behind its tight place, *12b*. This gentle pull will stretch the front top part of your left shoulder muscles. Hold this stretching position for 30 seconds to a minute.

Reverse this position by moving the triangle to your left and bending your left elbow. Use your left arm to pull your right extended arm back, *12c*. You should feel this stretch in the front of your right shoulder muscles. You may also feel the contraction of the muscles between your shoulder blades. Hold this stretch for 30 seconds to a minute.

Now extend your left arm. Return the triangle to be above your head. Carefully pull both arms completely back so that the rope is now behind your head and then behind your back, *12d*. Your extended but not locked arms will move backward and down, *12e,f,g*, so that the final position of your arms is down at your sides and the rope is behind you. If the preliminary stretches for each shoulder did not stretch your muscles enough to allow you to take your arms back comfortably, then move your hands a few inches apart on the rope and try again to bring the rope back. If you have very little difficulty the first time, decrease the space on the rope 1 to 2 inches and do this final stretch again. The final part of this stretch can be done lying on your bed on your back, with your head at the corner of the foot of the bed. In this position, when you take your arms over your head, gravity will help pull the weight of your arms and help stretch your muscles enough for them to yield and move through their full range of motion.

These shoulder muscle stretches, from below, from the side, and from above, are important to do before lifting weights, or playing tennis or any other racket sport. They are helpful for typists, pianists, bicyclists, painters and sculptors, writers, drummers, carpenters, and laborers. Anyone who uses his or her arms in a forward position can maintain flexibility and prevent stiffness and injury by using these stretches before and after work.

13

SNOW ANGEL

This exercise does two things: it stretches the muscles in the front of your shoulders and strengthens the muscles that hold your shoulder blades in place.

STARTING POSITION: Lie on your back. Bend your knees to make your lower back comfortable. Extend your arms out to your sides at shoulder height, palms up. Make sure to keep your shoulder blades down. *13a.*

THE STRENGTHENING EXERCISE: Lift up and hold your extended arms about 2 inches off the floor. Do not lock your elbows. Hold for 30 seconds. Now very slowly make one full circle with your arms just above the floor, taking 8 counts in one direction, and repeat, taking 8 counts in the other direction. The shape of the circle is more like an oval, about 10 inches around, *13b.* Repeat these two circles so you have completed four slow circles.

THE STRETCH: Rest your arms on the floor for 5 to 10 seconds. Enjoy the release of tension you feel in the front of your chest and shoulders. Now move your arms 6 inches up

13a
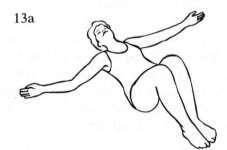

13b
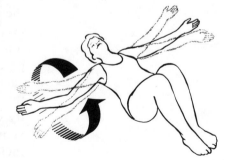

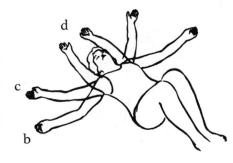

along the floor, pointing higher in a diagonal line out from your shoulders, *13c*. Repeat the sequence: lift, hold, 4 slow circles in alternating directions, and rest. Repeat this sequence again with your arms on a higher diagonal, and then once more with arms extended on the floor straight above your head, *13d*. During this entire exercise, make sure to keep your shoulder blades down. That will prevent your shoulders coming up too close to your ears. To make this exercise more challenging to your muscles, hold a shoe in each hand or hold a 1-pound can.

14   HUG THE WORLD

This exercise strengthens the muscles between your shoulder blades.

STARTING POSITION: Sit or stand. Be sure to align your head, lengthen your neck, relax your jaw, bring your shoulder blades down, and gently hold in your abdominal muscles. Reach both of your arms forward at shoulder height as though you were about to hug someone. Your palms are facing each other and are about 6 inches apart. *14a*.

THE STRENGTHENING EXERCISE: **(1)** Slowly bend your elbows while moving your extended arms toward your chest, *14b*. You should see your palms. Move your arms toward your chest so that your palms are about 4 to 6 inches from your chest. While you are doing step 1 you are **(2)** actively pulling your elbows sideways as though you could touch the walls on each side of you with your elbows, *14c*. Make sure to keep your shoulder blades pulling down.

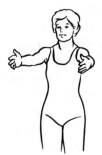

14a

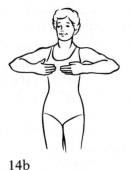

14b

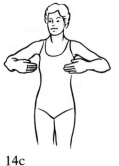

14c

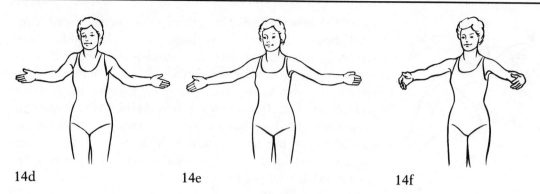

14d   14e   14f

(3) Slowly extend your forearms while at the same time trying to touch your elbows together behind your back, *14d*. You will feel the diamond-shaped muscle between your shoulder blades, the trapezius, contracting. Take 8 slow counts to do steps 1–3. To finish this exercise (4) pretend you are about to hug the world, or a big round object, in front of you and return your arms to the starting position, taking 4 slow counts, *14e,f*. If you do this last movement as though your arms were attached to a strong elastic behind you, you'll feel all the muscles on the palm side of your arm working. Repeat Hug the World three more times slowly. If you now do any of the shoulder stretches, you should feel your muscles stretch more easily.

15   CHICKEN

This exercise strengthens the downward depressors of your shoulder blades, the muscles between your shoulder blades, and the muscles on the back of your neck.

STARTING POSITION: Stand with your feet about 6 to 8 inches apart and pointing straight ahead. Now bend your knees deeply, as though you were about to sit on a low stool. Keep your heels on the floor. Let your entire upper body — pelvis, rib cage, and head — round forward so your lower back is parallel to the floor and the rest of your spine is rounded. The front of your torso, with your abdominal muscles held in, is very near your thighs. Your head is relaxed forward. The shape of your back and neck in this starting

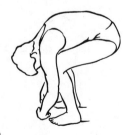

15a

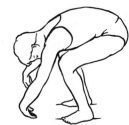

15b

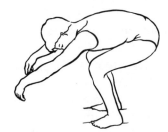

15c

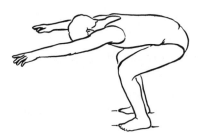

15d

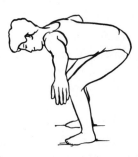

15e

position is like a turtle shell. Your arms are relaxed, hanging down toward the floor, *15a.*

THE STRENGTHENING EXERCISE: You are now going to slowly extend your spine from the rounded-down position into a straight line parallel to the floor. **(1)** Lift your rib cage in 2 counts, *15b,* and **(2)** then lift your arms to each side or straight ahead by closing your shoulder blades together, *15c,* or above your head by pulling your shoulder blades down. (You just felt the action of closing your shoulder blades together, a slow contraction, in exercise 14, Hug the World.) Raise your arms slowly, extended out to each side parallel to the floor, like open wings of a bird. Take 2 counts to do this. **(3)** Lift your neck in 2 counts and then **(4)** lift your head, *15d or e,* in 2 counts. Keep your face looking down at the floor; don't lift your head to see the wall in front of you, which would arch your neck. Now your spine is flat and your arms are reaching out to the sides. To complete this exercise, **(5)** lower your head in 2 counts, *15c;* **(6)** then lower your neck in 2 counts; **(7)** then lower your arms in 2 counts, *15b;* and **(8)** lower your rib cage in 2 counts, *15b.* You should now have returned to your starting position, *15a.* At no time during this exercise do you straighten your legs. Remaining in the bent-leg position protects your lower back.

Repeat this sequence with your arms reaching diagonally forward. Then repeat it with your arms reaching above your head, *15d,* and then with your arms reaching diagonally downward, *15e.*

There are two ways to make this exercise more challenging to your muscles. One way is to hold a shoe or a 1-pound weight (a can of applesauce will do) in each hand while doing the exercise. The other is to lift one leg and extend it out parallel to the floor. Do this by reaching back and out with the foot of the leg you are lifting. Do not straighten your one supporting leg; keep it bent in the original starting position. Press down the toes of your supporting leg to help keep yourself balanced.

{**Troubleshooting:** Here are three mistakes you may make in doing this exercise. **(1)** Don't only lift your arms and neglect to flatten out your upper back by forgetting to contract your shoulder blade muscles. **(2)** Don't initiate the action from your head and then end up arching your neck. Instead, start the movement from the bottom of your spine and flatten out from the bottom to the top, from your tail to your head. **(3)** When you try to lift your leg, along with the other parts of your body, complete the action and feel the muscles below your buttocks contract. Lift your leg parallel to the floor and don't let it droop.}

To stand up, bring your upper body upright before you straighten your legs. Hold in your abdominal muscles to start. Now tuck your buttocks under; this action will enable you to straighten up your torso. Standing in this bent-leg position tires your upper thigh muscles but also strengthens them.

{**Troubleshooting:** To protect yourself from knee strain during the exercise, make sure to keep your weight evenly distributed on the entire surface of your foot. Make sure to press your toes. Your knees may feel fatigued if your weight transfers forward, off your heels. Also, you may be bending your legs too much, so don't bend down quite so far. You may want to place your hands on your thighs to start lifting up your upper body.}

16   SHOULDER SHRUGS

This exercise can strengthen the downward depressors of your shoulder blades.

UP-DOWN

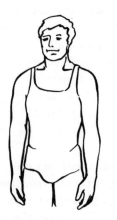

16a

STARTING POSITION: Sit or stand. Let your arms hang down at your sides, *16a*. Align your head, with your chin in and jaw relaxed. Make sure you have done the three shoulder stretches (exercises 10–12) so that throughout this exercise you can keep your shoulder blades gently pulled together and not rolled forward. This exercise is more effective if you hold a 1- or 2-pound weight in each hand.

THE STRENGTHENING EXERCISE: Hold a small weight in each hand and let your arms hang down by your sides. Do not lock your elbows and do not squeeze the weights in your hands. All the lifting and lowering should be done — you guessed it — slowly. **(1)** Lift your shoulders and then slowly pull them down so that you feel your front chest muscles causing this lowering movement to happen. Take 4 counts to lower your shoulders. **(2)** Lift up your shoulders and pull

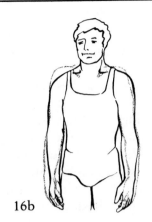
16b

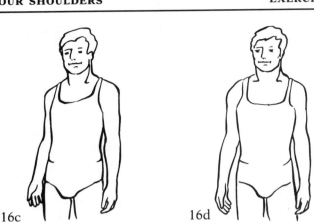
16c   16d

them down, feeling the muscles in back — the downward depressors of your shoulder blades — making this lowering movement happen, *16b*. Take 4 counts to do this. **(3)** Now lift up your shoulders in 4 counts and concentrate on feeling both groups of muscles in front and in back (the combination of steps 1 and 2) pull your shoulders down. **(4)** Finally, pretend you have a heavy weight on your shoulders and slowly lift it with your shoulders in 4 counts, and then lower your shoulders, feeling your front and back muscles causing the lowering movement to happen. Take 4 counts to do this. Repeat step 4 four more times.

You can move your shoulders forward and backward in the same manner. To move your shoulder forward, concentrate on contracting the front muscles while extending the back ones, and vice versa. Your shoulders start in place and move one at a time. **(1)** Contract the muscles in front and pull your shoulder into a rounded position. Feel the front muscles contract while the back ones relax. Take 2 counts to do this. **(2)** Bring your shoulder back to place by contracting the muscles between your shoulder blades. Take 2 counts to do this. **(3)** Pull your shoulder back in 2 counts and feel the muscles between your shoulder blades contract and your front muscles relax, *16c*. **(4)** Return your shoulder to the centered starting position by slowly relaxing the contraction between your shoulder blades a little, *16d*. Take 2 counts to do this. Repeat the sequence of steps 1–4 with the other shoulder. Now try both shoulders at the same time. Do it slowly.

17   SHOULDER CIRCLES

These circles are a combination of the up-down and for-ward-back exercises you just finished. Pay careful attention to each group of muscles you use when doing these circles. First work with each shoulder separately before doing both at the same time. **(1)** Start by bringing your shoulder for-ward, taking 2 counts. **(2)** Lift up your shoulder as though lifting something heavy, taking 2 counts. **(3)** Pull your shoulder back in 2 counts and **(4)** pull it down and relax into the beginning position in 2 counts. Reverse the direction of the circle: back, up, forward, down. Feel each position in your muscles. Try this shoulder circle with the other shoulder, and then try circling both shoulders at the same time. If you do this faster, to the tick of a clock, continue to concentrate on feeling your muscles do the movements. Don't let momentum take over, because then you will mainly be exercising your ligaments, and that is not your goal.

18   HANGING FROM A BAR

You learned in the anatomy section that the downward depressors of our shoulder blades are weak because we don't hang from trees the way primates do. Therefore, to strengthen these muscles we need to practice hanging from trees. In order to do this exercise you need a bar to hang from: you can use a chinning bar, or a secure basement pipe, or a school yard jungle gym or monkey bars. Test the strength of the bar before you do this exercise. If you already have the strength to do chin-ups, then you should do them. You do not have to just hang. See the instructions at the end of this exercise.

STARTING POSITION: Place your hands on the bar with your palms forward. Align your head straight up, chin in, jaw relaxed. Put your feet forward about 8 to 10 inches; they should not be straight down underneath your pelvis. This forward position of your legs guards your back against arching when you hang from the bar.

THE STRENGTHENING EXERCISE: Bend your knees and

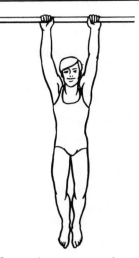

18a   (wrong starting position)

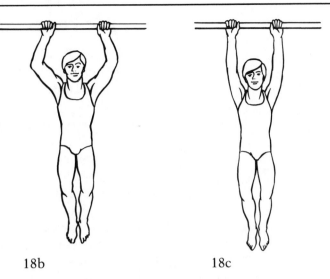

18b   18c

hang from your hands. Do not lock your elbows, and don't let your shoulder blades come up, *18a*. Contract your abdominal muscles and hold them in while you lift your knees up a little off the floor. Hang with your feet off the floor and try to bend your elbows to pull yourself up as though you were going to touch your head to the bar, *18b*. The action of hanging and supporting your weight will strengthen the muscles that keep your shoulder blades down and together, *18c*. See how long you can hold your feet off the floor. Try 4 to 6 counts. Rest your feet on the floor and then lift your knees and hold again. Repeat this for a total of four times. As you get stronger, lengthen the number of holding counts to 8 and then to 10. Continue to try to lift yourself up toward the bar.

To do chin-ups, slowly lift yourself up to touch the top of your head, and eventually your chin, to the bar, *18b*. Take 4 slow counts to lift up and 4 counts to lower your body down. When you finish, stretch out your wrists and shoulder muscles, using the stretches in the beginning of this chapter and the next (exercises 20–22).

19   LIFTING FROM YOUR CHAIR

This exercise is to strengthen the downward depressors of your shoulder blades by having you lift your body weight from below. Hanging from a Bar (exercise 18) strengthens them by having you lift your weight from above.

STARTING POSITION: Sit on a dining room or kitchen chair with or without arms. Place your hands at your sides, on the seat or on the arms of the chair. Place your lower legs straight down from your knees so your feet are about 6 to 10 inches in front of the chair, *19a*. During this exercise, make sure to keep your shoulder blades down and back.

THE STRENGTHENING EXERCISE: (1) Slowly lift yourself up from the seat in a vertical direction, taking 4 counts. Keep your feet on the floor. **(2)** Hold this position for 4 counts. **(3)** Slowly lower your body down to the seat of the chair, *19b*. Repeat steps 1–3 five more times. You will feel this exercise in your hands, forearms, and upper arms. If you start and do this exercise with your shoulder blades down, you will also be strengthening your downward depressors.

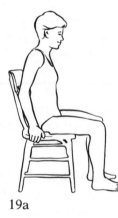

19a

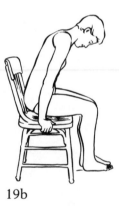

19b

6 Your Arms

Anatomy

When you move your entire arm, you use the bones, joints, and muscles of your shoulder girdle. Because your arms also have elbow and wrist joints, you can use your arms without your shoulders' contributing to the movement. This chapter focuses on stretching and strengthening exercises for your arms, but you know that you will use your shoulders and hands to do them. The division of your body into these parts is only for the convenience of describing their workings in detail.

The structure of your arms enables you to use your hands in their many thousands of ways and to carry out these actions without thinking *(VI-A)*. Three cheers for your arm joints: your shoulders, your elbows, and your wrists. The lower end of your upper arm bone, the humerus, joins your two forearm bones, the radius and ulna, at your elbow. These forearm bones join the end of your humerus in a side-by-side position. The bone that you lean on when you rest your elbow on the table is the ulna. Together your radius and ulna flex and extend, bend and straighten. The structure of your elbow joint does not permit your forearm to move side to side. The reason you can swat flies or draw a circle with your arm bent is that your upper arm moves at your shoulder.

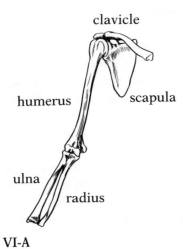

clavicle

humerus

scapula

ulna

radius

VI-A

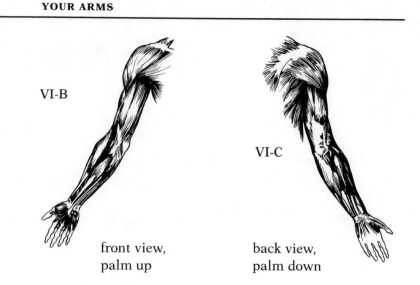

VI-B

VI-C

front view,
palm up

back view,
palm down

You can turn your hand over so your palm is up or turn your hand so your palm is down because your radius rotates or rolls over your ulna. Put one of your hands around your other forearm and turn your palm up and down to feel how this works. You can bend and straighten your forearm and rotate it without using your shoulder by keeping your upper arm in one position, and you can move your forearm in all these ways while you are moving your upper arm too because your shoulder muscles cooperate with the rest of your arm. Like your other joints, your elbow and wrist are bound together with ligaments.

The muscles of your arm are arranged to enable you to do all these wonderful movements in endless combinations. Your arm flexors are the most popular muscles to show when someone says to you, "Show me your muscles." You flex your forearm and show them your biceps. These muscles are located on the front of your upper arm and attach below your elbow to lift your forearm and to make this bent-arm movement possible *(VI-B)*. The muscles on the back of your upper arm, the triceps, extend your forearm *(VI-C)*. You also have muscles that turn your palm down, that is, pronate your forearm and hand; and you have muscles called supinators that turn your palm up. These are located primarily on your forearm and rotate your radius and ulna in the coordinated way that you have come to expect.

Weight lifting is increasingly common now for women as well as men. When you think of weight lifting, you usually think of building arm strength primarily for your upper arms, though weights are made for strengthening all your muscle groups. You don't have to lift weights if you want to build, maintain, or increase your arms' capacity to lift, move, or hold. You can use chin-ups for your biceps and push-ups for your triceps, the muscles on the backs of your upper arms. In the traditionally fast style, push-ups are strenuous and hard for beginners to do. This chapter contains beginner forms of these exercises and all of them are done slowly.

One of the major problems for this part of your body is muscle imbalance. This comes from poor posture and from not stretching the arm and shoulder muscles involved in daily front-reaching activities. Chronic difficulties in shoulder, elbow, and neck often result from these imbalances.

Arm strengthening exercises, especially when done fast, make these imbalances worse and can cause muscle strains and even tears. Injuries can occur in your shoulders from not having your shoulder blades down and back during an entire exercise; in your elbows from locking them; and in your wrists from not pressing your fingers. Pressing your fingers prevents straining your wrist ligaments when you passively rest on your wrists.

Wrist, hand, and finger exercises are found in Chapter 7. The care of tennis elbow is described in Chapter 16.

Exercises

Your arm and shoulder muscles are working during all the exercises in this chapter. They emphasize the groups of muscles in your upper and lower arm and also train their coordination. The exercises in Chapter 7, "Your Wrists, Hands, and Fingers," will also involve the muscles in your arms.

20

TRICEPS STRETCH

The shoulder stretches (exercises 10–12) in Chapter 5 stretch some of the muscles in your arms, wrists, and forearms. There is another area of your arm that you need to stretch — your triceps.

STARTING POSITION: Stand 18 to 24 inches from a wall, and turn so your right side faces the wall. Reach your right arm up and place the little finger side of your hand and your entire forearm on the wall. Your palm is forward, not on the wall. The direction of your arm from your body is a high diagonal to the side. *20a.*

THE STRETCH: Now lean a little on your forearm. To feel more stretch, slide it up the wall a little, *20b.* You should feel a stretch in the back part of your upper arm. You may need to turn your entire body a little bit to the left to feel the stretch. Hold that position for 30 seconds to a minute. Repeat the stretch on your left arm.

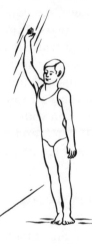

20a   20b

21

WRIST STRETCH

This stretch also belongs in Chapter 7, "Your Wrists, Hands, and Fingers," but it is here because your forearms need this stretch now. You can do this stretch after any activity in

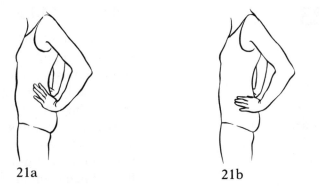

21a   21b

which you hold on to something for a long time, such as a hammer, a tennis racket, or bike handlebars, or when you keep your fingers curved, as in typing, writing, or playing the piano, guitar, violin, or harp.

STARTING POSITION: Bend your hands back at the wrist and place them on the back of your hips, right below your waist. Try to place your palms against your hips, and keep your fingers up, *21a*, or pointing forward with your wrists together, *21b*. Keep your shoulder blades down and back.

THE STRETCH: By putting your hands in either of these positions, you can feel a stretch in your forearms, wrists, and fingers. Hold them there for 30 seconds to a minute. Move your hand so you can put more pressure on your thumb, and then on your little finger. This position stretches the forearm muscles much more than just pulling your hand back with the other hand.

---

22   FOREARM STRETCH

This stretch loosens the tight muscles on the top part of your forearm. It is very simple.

THE STRETCH: Bend your hands forward at the wrist with your fingers extended and together. Extend your arms forward or to your sides and rotate your arms down and back. This arm rotation turns your elbows up. To feel the stretch you must keep your wrist bent. Hold this position for 30 seconds to a minute. Once you feel the stretch, keep your arms in the same position and reverse the bend of your wrists. That is, bend them back and continue to feel the stretch.

23

ARM CIRCLES

Fast arm circles, both horizontal and vertical, are frequently part of warm-up sequences. They can be mild arm strengthening exercises if you slow them down. If you hold a 1- or 3-pound weight in each hand, Arm Circles will be more challenging.

HORIZONTAL

STARTING POSITION: You can sit or stand. When sitting, align your head, with your chin in and jaw relaxed. Hold in your abdominal muscles and place your feet firmly on the floor. When standing, align your upper body this same way and unlock your knees in order to keep your lower back relaxed. Place your feet straight forward and press your toes down. Extend your arms sideways at shoulder height and take care to keep your elbows unlocked throughout the entire exercise. *23a.*

THE STRENGTHENING EXERCISE: **(1)** Slowly draw a circle about 8 inches in circumference, starting forward and up, *23b.* Take 8 slow counts to do this. **(2)** Draw another circle in the reverse direction, starting down and back. Take 8 slow counts to do this. Repeat these circles three more times in each direction for a total of 8 slow circles. When you finish Arm Circles, stretch your muscles by doing the shoulder stretches from below or from the side (exercises 10,11).

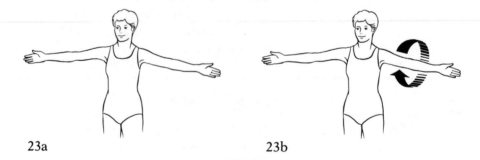

23a   23b

VERTICAL

Vertical Arm Circles are a variation of the horizontal ones. The starting position is the same, except your arms will start down at your sides. Be sure to keep your shoulders down and back and your elbows unlocked.

THE STRENGTHENING EXERCISE: **(1)** Very slowly circle one arm and then the other up, forward, back, and down.

Take 20 counts to do this. **(2)** Reverse the direction of your first circle and start back, up, forward, and down. Take 20 slow counts to do this. Repeat these circles three more times in each direction for a total of 8 slow circles. Holding a 1-or 3-pound weight in your hands makes this more challenging. When you finish, make sure to stretch out your shoulder muscles as above.

24   **CUTTING CHEESE**

STARTING POSITION: You can sit or stand for this exercise. Let your arms hang down at your sides. Align your head and keep your shoulder blades back and down during the entire process of lifting and lowering your arms. This will not be easy to do because your shoulders automatically lift and therefore can roll forward whenever you lift your arm. You have to make a conscious effort to keep your shoulder blades in place. This exercise will be more effective if you hold a 1-pound weight or can in each hand. *24a.*

THE STRENGTHENING EXERCISE: Your arms will lift out to each side with your palms down. **(1)** Slowly lift your arms up as high as they will go, *24b.* Take 8 counts to do this. Imagine that the top surface of your arm is a cheese cutter and that you are cutting upward through cheese. This image is to get you to feel resistance as you lift your arms. **(2)** Now

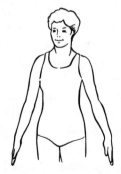

24a

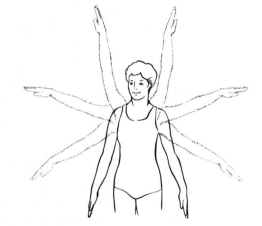

24b

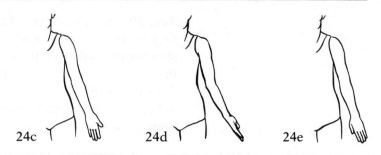

24c   24d   24e

lower your arms as if cutting through cheese, pushing down with the entire surface of each arm, palm down. Take 8 counts to do this. Allow your arms to rest hanging down. **(3)** Now rotate your arm so that your palms are forward, *24c.* Slowly lift up your arms as high as they will go. You should be able to raise them higher than in step 1. When you lift your arms, you will be "cutting cheese" with your thumb up and your little finger down. In this position, you should feel a different sensation in your arm muscles than you felt in steps 1 and 2. Take 8 counts to do this. **(4)** Now lower your arms with resistance as though cutting through cheese or pressing down a gigantic spring. Allow your arms to rest, hanging down. **(5)** Rotate your arms again, this time trying to put your little fingers forward, *24d.* When you lift your arms this time, the surface pressing up is the palm sides of your hands and arms, the inside surfaces. Slowly lift your arms as high as they will go. Take 8 counts to do this. Again in this position, as in steps 3 and 4, your arm will rise higher than in steps 1 and 2. **(6)** Slowly lower your arms, pushing or pressing down with the entire surface of your arms. Do not lock your elbows. Take 8 counts to do this. Allow your arms to rest down at your sides. **(7)** Now rotate your arms in so that your thumb is near your side and your little finger is out, *24e.* The other two rotations, thumb up (3 and 4) and palm up (5 and 6), were outward rotations. Your little finger will be up and your thumb down as you cut through cheese this time. Slowly lift your arm, feeling the elbow surface of your arm pressing up. Lift your arms as high as they will go. In this position, as in step 1, your arms do not go as high as in steps 3 and 4 and steps 5 and 6. **(8)** Slowly lower your arms as if pressing down a giant spring. Take care to keep your shoulder blades back. Allow your arms to rest.

VARIATIONS

This exercise can be done with your arms reaching out in front of you, or behind you, or diagonally to the front or back. You should rotate your arm so each of the four surfaces leads for each lifting pathway.

You can also do this lying on your back on the floor. Bend your knees enough that the bottoms of your feet are on the floor, to relax your lower back. Then when you lift your arms, holding 1- or 3-pound weights, make sure to keep your shoulder blades down. You may find that using one arm at a time is easier to control. **(1)** Your arms will lift slightly off the floor and remain parallel to it when your pathway starts with your arms down and hover close to the floor as your arm's pathway creates a half circle. This is like making Snow Angels (exercise 13). During the other front and diagonal pathways, your arms will come off the floor and up to a vertical position. Your starting positions will be: **(2)** arms down at your sides; **(3)** arms out to your sides; **(4)** arms above your head; **(5)** arms at a low diagonal; and **(6)** arms on a high diagonal. For each pathway, lift your arms as far as they will go, keeping your shoulder blades down. When you have finished this entire exercise, stretch the muscles you just used with stretches for your shoulders (exercises 10–12), arms (exercises 20–22), and wrists (exercises 33–36).

25   BEGINNER'S PUSH-UPS

STARTING POSITION: Kneel on all fours on the floor. Be sure your arms are straight down from your shoulders. Do not lock your elbows. Open your fingers, point them forward or slightly out, and press them down firmly. Extend your feet so the tops are on the floor. Make sure your feet reach straight back; don't let them turn in or out. This foot position gives your knees comfort and protects them. Walk your hands forward about 10 to 12 inches. This change in your "all fours" position will take your thighs out of the perpendicular and move them into a forward diagonal line, *25a*. Another way to get into this starting position is to put your body into the position for regular Push-ups (exercise 26) and then gently put your knees down on the floor.

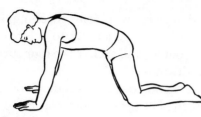

25a

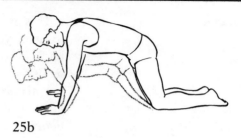

25b

THE STRENGTHENING EXERCISE: **(1)** Slowly bend your elbows and lower your body. Take 4 counts to do this. **(2)** Lift your body by slowly straightening your arms in 4 counts, *25b*. Repeat this sequence four to six times. When you find that these push-ups get easy, then you are ready for regular Push-ups.

26 PUSH-UPS

STARTING POSITION: Kneel on all fours on the floor. Place your arms straight down from your shoulders. Do not lock your elbows. Open your fingers, point them forward or slightly out, and press them down firmly. Align your head straight out from your shoulders, relax your jaw, and don't grit your teeth while you do this exercise. Extend your legs back and hold your body up so that your buttocks are up and out of line with the rest of your body, *26a*. This position of your pelvis takes the strain off your lower back. Hold in your abdominal muscles. Also keep your knees relaxed; do not lock them. Keep your feet 4 to 6 inches apart.

THE STRENGTHENING EXERCISE: **(1)** Slowly bend your elbows to lower your body. Take 4 counts to do this. Bend your elbows no farther than where you can still control the motion, *26b*. **(2)** Slowly extend your arms to lift your body

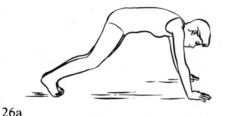

26a

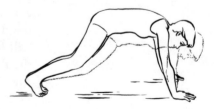

26b

back up. Take 4 counts to do this. Do not lock your elbows when you complete this lifting. Repeat this lowering and lifting movement four to six more times. If you want it to be more challenging, then slow down the lowering and lifting, taking 6 or even 8 counts.

27

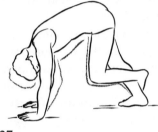

27a

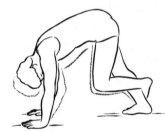

27b

A-FRAME PUSH-UPS

This modification of regular Push-ups (exercise 26) is used by runners to enable them to push off fast at the beginning of a race. The deltoid muscle at the top and in front of your shoulder gets strengthened in this position. The only difference between the A-frame Push-up and the regular one is the starting position.

STARTING POSITION: To make the A, get into the position for regular Push-ups and then reach your buttocks up and move your hands about 12 inches closer to your feet. Your body will fold where your legs insert into their hip sockets. Keep your back straight and abdominal muscles held in, place your unlocked arms straight down from your shoulders, and extend your head so it is in line with your spine, *27a*. Don't lift up your head and arch your neck, and don't lower your head below your arms, which will misalign the vertebrae in your neck. The foot position of this push-up gives your calf muscles a strong stretch. As in A-frame Calf Stretch (exercise 87) rest the front of one foot on the heel of the other, or place one foot on the floor forward of the leg you are stretching first, and do two push-ups. Change feet and do two more.

THE STRENGTHENING EXERCISE: **(1)** Slowly bend your elbows to lower your body, *27b*. Take 4 counts to do this. Lower yourself only to where you feel your arm muscles controlling the movement. Don't drop into your elbows. **(2)** Slowly extend your arms and lift yourself back up in 4 counts. Repeat this four to six more times. {**Troubleshooting:** If you allow your heel to come off the floor too far, your entire body will move forward, not just down and up. Only lower and raise your body in the down-and-up pathway.}

Stretch your shoulder muscles when you finish doing any of these push-ups (see Chapter 5).

28

TWO ARM

FRONT WALL PUSH-UPS

These push-ups are good for beginners to start to gain arm strength.

READYING POSITION: Stand near a wall. Keep your head aligned so your ears are over your shoulders, chin in, and jaw relaxed. Keep your shoulder blades down and gently hold in your abdominal muscles. Keep your knees unlocked and your feet straight ahead.

STARTING POSITION: Face the wall and stand an arm's length away from it. Place your palms on the wall with your fingers up. Angle your upper body so it bends forward at the hips, *28a*. This body alignment, as in regular Push-ups (exercise 26), protects your lower back.

THE STRENGTHENING EXERCISE: **(1)** Slowly bend your elbows and lean into the wall, *28b*. (Your elbows bend down toward the floor.). Only go in as far as your arms can control the weight of your body. Your entire body is slowly leaning in toward the wall. Take 4 slow counts to do this. **(2)** Now push your body back away from the wall by slowly straightening your elbows. Take 4 slow counts to do this. {**Troubleshooting:** Make sure to keep leaning your weight forward onto your hands when you begin straightening your arms. Otherwise you will use momentum to come away from the wall.}

Repeat this Wall Push-up ten times. If this seems too easy, slow down the counts and take 6 counts to go in toward the wall and 6 counts to push away from it. As you move toward and away from the wall, you will feel mild stretching in your calf muscles (see Chapter 13).

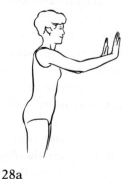

28a

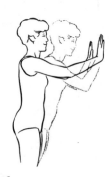

28b

ONE ARM

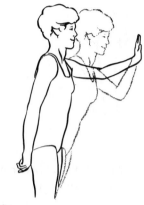

28c

Use this exercise if one of your arms is weaker than the other. Follow all the instructions for two-arm Wall Push-ups, except first put your left arm down at your side and center your right arm on the wall between the spots where you placed both of your palms. **(1)** Slowly bend your elbow and lean toward the wall, taking 4 slow counts. Your elbow points diagonally down toward the floor, *28c*. **(2)** Slowly push back away from the wall by straightening your elbow. Be careful not to lock your elbow when you finish extending your arm. Repeat this six to ten times. Now repeat this exercise with your left arm six to ten times. You can alternate arms every time, or every other time, or after four to six repetitions. Or repeat ten times with each arm.

A much more challenging way to do this is to place your arm directly in front of your shoulder instead of centering it in front of your chest. As you do this variation, be careful to keep your body from twisting or having the shoulder of the nonworking arm fall in toward the wall. You need to keep your body at a right angle to your working arm. Keep your body squarely facing the wall. Repeat with the other arm. Use the same slow 4 to 6 counts in and 4 to 6 counts out. Stretch your arms after you finish this exercise, using shoulder stretches (exercises 10–12).

29

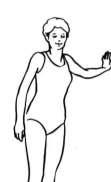

29a

SIDE WALL PUSH-UPS

The readying position directions for these push-ups are the same as for Front Wall Push-ups.

STARTING POSITION: Stand an arm's length away from a wall with your side toward the wall. The front of your body is at a right angle to the wall. (This starting position is the same as for Shoulder Stretch from the Side, exercise 11.) Put your hand on the wall with your fingers up, *29a*. Keep pressing all your fingers during the entire exercise.

THE STRENGTHENING EXERCISE: **(1)** Slowly bend your elbow and lean your entire body, held straight, toward the wall. Only lean in as far as you can without losing control of the movement with your arm muscles, *29b*. Do not go so far that you tightly fold (overbend) your elbow. Take 4 slow

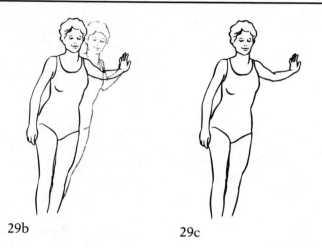

29b   29c

counts to do this. **(2)** Now slowly push your body away from the wall by straightening your elbow. Take 4 slow counts to do this. Repeat this bending and straightening six to ten times.

This exercise is very useful for strengthening the downward depressors of your shoulder blades. To feel this effect, you need to adjust the starting position of these push-ups. Instead of standing with your body at a right angle to the wall, you need to turn your body slightly so that your back is toward the wall at a small angle, *29c*. Don't turn as far as you did to feel the Shoulder Stretch from the Side. Only turn your body enough so that when you do these push-ups, you can feel the muscles below your shoulder blade working. Repeat this exercise on your other arm. Finish by doing the Shoulder Stretch from the Side.

Coordination Exercises

When you try to imitate the way seagulls, cormorants, and mallards use their wings when they fly, the resulting fluidity of movement and control you gain helps you to coordinate all the parts of your arms and, of course, strengthens the muscles you use while doing these movements.

30

SEAGULLS

READYING POSITION: This position is exactly the same as the others in this chapter. Your head needs to be held vertically, your ears need to be over your shoulders, your chin in, your jaw relaxed, your shoulder blades held down, and your abdominal muscles held in.

STARTING POSITION: You can sit or stand. Let your arms hang down close to your sides. If you sit on the floor, your arms should not be resting on the floor.

THE COORDINATION EXERCISE: **(1)** Slowly begin to open a space under your armpits as though a balloon were slowly blowing up under your arms, *30*. As the space between your arms and sides enlarges, you will lift each part of your upper arms, then your elbows, then your forearms, then your wrists, the tops of your hands, and then your fingers. Each part opens out in sequence away from your body about 3 to 6 inches. The space of your moving arms is curved like the handle of a teacup. The end shape is a long diagonal line starting at your armpits. Take 4 slow counts to do this. **(2)** Just at the moment that your arms extend into a straight line, you will begin to close the space at your armpits. To do this, push your elbows down and in toward your sides. You will need to rotate your elbows from their lifted position and point them down. This will cause your forearms, wrists, and hands to sweep up a little more than their final diagonal line, before these parts of your arms begin to close in toward your sides. Take 4 slow counts to do this. When you have closed your arms down to the starting position, immediately start the opening process again. Repeat this three more times and then try to do it faster, while continuing to feel

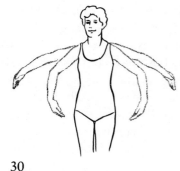

30

your arm muscles controlling the movements. Don't let your arms just flop. Seagulls can also be done with your arms reaching forward and backward. You can also allow your arms to rise to extend horizontally out to your sides instead of only moving them in a vertical position. Take four repetitions of Seagulls to move from a vertical position into a horizontal one.

31   CORMORANTS

STARTING POSITION: Lift your arms out to your sides horizontally at shoulder height and have your palms facing forward so your thumbs are up and your little fingers are down, *31a.*

THE COORDINATION EXERCISE: **(1)** While holding your upper arms completely still, slowly fold your forearms forward. Take 4 counts to do this. Your forearms may move beyond a 90 degree angle toward one as small as 45 degrees but this is not necessary. *31b,c.* **(2)** Slowly extend your forearms to the starting position. Take 4 counts to do this. Repeat this exercise three more times. The challenge of this exercise is to keep your upper arms from moving at all. Try to keep them entirely still during both parts of this exercise, the closing and opening of your forearms. You can vary this exercise by folding your forearms down or up. These variations require only that you change the starting positions of your hands and forearms. Be sure to keep your upper arms still and don't allow your shoulder blades to come forward.

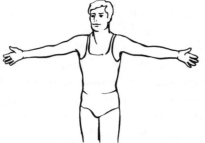

31a

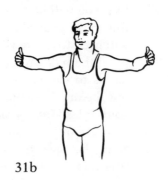

31b

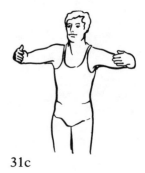

31c

32

MALLARDS

Have you ever looked up in the sky and seen a flock of ducks? Their wings appear to move up and down from the place where they attach to their bodies. They flap their wings without bending at the equivalent to our elbow joint. In this next coordination exercise, you will try to move your arms the way mallards use their wings in flight.

STARTING POSITION: Sit or stand with your arms extended horizontally out to your sides at shoulder height. Keep your elbows unlocked and your wrists and fingers extended.

THE COORDINATION EXERCISE: **(1)** Slowly close the entire length of your arms toward each other until they are extended out in front of you. Move each arm as one long unit and imagine that you are flying against stiff wind resistance, *32a,b*. Take 4 slow counts to do this. **(2)** Now open your arms and retrace the path you just made. Pass your starting point and open your arms behind you as far as they will go, while keeping your shoulder blades down and your arms on the same level as they began, at shoulder height, *32c*. Take 4 slow counts to do this. Continue to move your arms from back to front and front to back four to six more times.

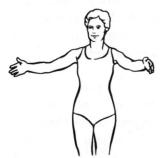

32a

32b

32c

When you build enough strength to do these coordination exercises smoothly, you can try to hold 1-pound weights in each hand or attach weights to your wrists. Be sure to stretch your shoulder, arm, and wrist muscles when you complete these exercises.

7 Your Wrists, Hands, and Fingers

VII-A

Anatomy

You would have a hard time reading this book if it were not for your hands. The complex and magnificently coordinated structure of your hands makes you able to do distinctly human activities, such as eat with a knife and fork, write, type, pick up tiny objects, thread a needle, or perform microsurgery. These activities depend on your hands' responding to commands from your brain. The bones, their ligaments, and the muscles in your hands allow you to do almost anything you want to do.

You have twenty-seven bones in each of your hands — that's a lot of bones to have in such a small area of your body! These bones and their joints give your hands their mobility and dexterity *(VII-A)*. Your arm bones join your hands at the wrist. Your wrists have eight bones, in two rows of four bones each. The first row of bones connects your hand to your arm and the second row of bones attaches to the five bones in your palm. These five palm bones are longer versions of your finger bones. You can feel and see the shape of these because each of your fingers is a separate unit made up of three more similar bones, in shorter and shorter form. Your thumbs also have three bones, but they are positioned differently in your hands, primarily so that your thumbs can reach each of your other fingers — the important "opposable" function.

The ligaments that hold all these bones together are, in many cases, looser than others in your body because the looseness allows your hands the mobility they need. Your eight wrist bones are in a low bridgelike shape. The ligaments that bind your wrist bones together maintain a small tunnel to let nerves, tendons, and muscles pass under it. The joint capsules, which are ligaments and tissue that hold each of your many hand and finger joints together, are also loose where you need to bend your fingers and thumbs.

Because you use your hands all the time, you know the range of movement that they have. Your wrists move up, down, and side to side, and a combination of these movements allows you to move your wrists around clockwise and counterclockwise. By using your fingers, you can fold your palm in from the sides and flatten it again. Your fingers can make a fist, curve, or flex; and unfist, straighten out, or extend. They can also separate, spread apart like a fan opening, close together, and even overlap or bundle together. They can move separately or in concert. They can each make circles in any direction. Your thumbs can do all this and touch all of your other fingers. Your thumbs' mobility is the primary reason that your hands can accomplish all their miraculous achievements.

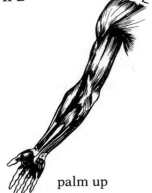

VII-B

palm up

Your hands have many muscles to allow you to move your bones around in this wide variety of directions *(VII-B)*. Your arm muscles provide your wrists their mobility. So do your finger muscles. The muscles in your palms move your wrists and your fingers. Some of your finger muscles start on your forearms and some of them start in your palms. The muscles that flex your fingers are stronger and more abundant than those that extend them. Your thumbs have eight (some anatomists say nine) muscles to let you move them in so many ways. All these muscles need a balance of stretch and strength to keep moving efficiently and effectively.

Since your hands are structured for grasping and climbing, they work better in certain positions than others. You have probably discovered the hard way that your fingers cannot grasp as strongly when your wrists are flexed, that is, bent forward, very far. You may also have discovered that your wrists can provide your arms more stability when your fingers are not holding or doing something. Then they can remain relaxed or actively help you stabilize your arms. Most of the time your muscles adjust automatically to the task you are doing, but it should help you to know how to use your hands in the most advantageous positions.

The way you use your hands determines how stretched and strong they are. Unless you give your hand muscles a wide variety of movements, they will gradually lose their natural range of motion. Here is an example to illustrate this idea. Make a fist and hold it for 30 seconds. Now relax your grip. What happens to your fingers? Do they uncurl to their extended position? Probably not, unless you deliberately open your hand and stretch out your fingers. So even the way you relax your hands influences how strong and stretched your hand muscles are. By doing the exercises in this chapter you will enable your hands to remain the mechanical miracle that they are. These exercises also enable you to regain lost flexibility and dexterity caused by lack of use, injury, and some joint diseases.

Exercises

READYING POSITION: Though you will now be concentrating only on your wrists, hands, and fingers, you will need to put your neck, shoulders, and abdominal muscles on "automatic pilot" and keep your head aligned, your shoulders down and back, and your abdominal muscles held in. The wrist rotation exercises may be easier to do if you are sitting at a desk or table where you can rest your elbows.

33   WRIST CIRCLES

In these exercises, the stretching and strengthening are simultaneous; that is, when you contract and strengthen muscles on the tops of your wrists, you will be stretching the muscles on the palm sides of your hands and vice versa.

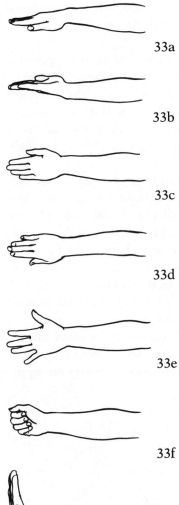

33a

33b

33c

33d

33e

33f

33g

STARTING POSITION: You can do this wrist exercise in four starting positions: palms down, *33a;* palms up, *33b;* thumbs up, *33c;* and thumbs down with little fingers up, *33d.* You can also do this with your fingers extended and spread apart, *33e,* or extended and closed together, *33a,* or with your hand held in a gentle, relaxed fist, *33f.* The directions will be in detail for one palm position. You can repeat the exercise putting your hand in the other three starting positions.

THE EXERCISE: Hold your hand straight out so there is no bend at your wrists, *33a.* **(1)** Slowly lift up your fingers, closed together, toward the top of your forearms. Do this by contracting the muscles on top of your wrist, *33g,* taking 4 counts. **(2)** Slowly press your hands down to the starting position, *33a,* taking 4 slow counts. **(3)** Now press your hands down, trying to put your palms at a right angle to your forearms. Keep your fingers extended straight from palms, *33h,* taking 4 slow counts. **(4)** Slowly lift your hands back up to the straight ahead starting position, *33a,* in 4 slow counts. **(5)** Now move your hands to the side by trying to close your little fingers to the sides of your forearms, *33i.* Do this in 4 slow counts. **(6)** Return your hands to the straight-ahead starting position, *33a,* in 4 slow counts. **(7)** Move your hands sideways by trying to close your thumbs to the side of your forearms, *33j.* Do this in 4 slow counts. **(8)** Return your hands to their starting position, *33a.*

Repeat this sequence — up, flat, down, flat, side, center, side, center — with your fingers open wide apart and then make a relaxed fist and repeat this sequence without using your finger muscles. Repeat this sequence three more times. In a new starting position for your wrist, each sequence has three parts, the first with your fingers extended and closed, the second with fingers open, and the third with your fingers gently curled in a fist.

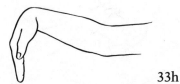

33h

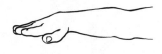

33i   33j

77

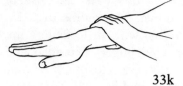

33k

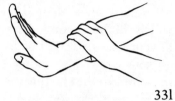

33l

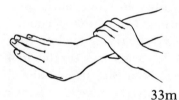

33m

To complete this wrist exercise, you will trace a circle with your hand and incorporate all the separate directions that you did in the first parts.

STARTING POSITION: Begin in the first starting position with your hands extended, palms down, fingers closed together. Place your elbows on a desk or table. This will help you stabilize your forearms in each of the starting positions so that you will use mainly your wrist muscles. Normally, to move your wrist, your forearm and wrist muscles coordinate. *33k.*

THE EXERCISE: **(1)** Lift your hands up, *33l;* **(2)** rotate them out to the little finger side, *33m,n;* **(3)** fold them down, *33o,p;* and **(4)** move them sideways to the thumb side of your hands, *33q,r.* **(5)** Lift your hand up so your wrist is bent and your fingers are up, *33l;* and **(6)** return them to the flat starting position, *33g.* Take 8 slow counts to do each circle. Now reverse the direction of your circle. Repeat these circles with your fingers open and then with your fingers curled in a fist. You can now use the other starting positions to repeat these circles. Take care to anchor each arm with the other in each new starting position to maintain your palms up, thumbs up, and thumbs down. Stretch out your wrist by doing the Forearm Stretch (exercise 22).

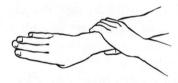

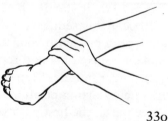

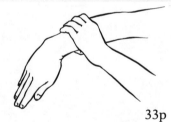

33n   33o   33p

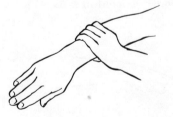

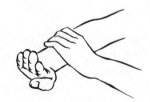

33q   33r

34

HAND TWISTS

As you get older, your hands seem to lose their mobility and dexterity. If you balance stretching with strengthening this is much less likely to occur. In this wrist exercise, you use your wrist muscles in a way you do not usually use them. By keeping your muscles mobile, you will be able to count on their dexterity when you need it.

STARTING POSITION: Sit where you can rest your elbows on a desk or table. Hold your forearms forward, up and off the table, bent at the elbows, palms down. Keep your fingers closed together and extended.

THE EXERCISE: **(1)** Slowly turn your hands over so your palms are toward the ceiling, and continue to turn your hand as if it could keep turning. You are trying to have your little fingers turn up toward and be parallel to the ceiling. Do this in 4 slow counts. **(2)** Now turn your hand back down and try to keep turning it as though you could twist your little fingers up to the ceiling. Take 4 slow counts to do this. Pretend you are pushing something or lifting something up, and then pressing it down. Repeat this with your fingers stretched apart and extended but not locked. Then repeat this sequence of turning over and back three more times each, with your extended fingers closed and then open. You may also want to do this exercise with your fingers loosely held in a fist. With your fingers held gently curled, you will feel a different sensation in your wrist than when you do this exercise with your fingers extended.

35

FINGER FAN

STARTING POSITION: Hang your arms comfortably down at your sides. Bend your arms and hold your forearms forward, palms down. Extend your fingers.

THE EXERCISE: **(1)** Slowly open your fingers wide apart, as though you had a tight rubber band wrapped around your fingers. Take 4 counts to do this. **(2)** Slowly close your fingers together as though there were tight springs between your fingers and the springs kept your fingers apart. Take 4 counts to do this. **(3)** Now curve your palms and fingers as though a large baseball were being pressed into your hand. Actively press your hands and fingers onto this imaginary baseball, *35a*. **(4)** Slowly flatten your hand into your first extended position, *35b*, taking 4 slow counts. Now turn your hands over and repeat this sequence of open and close, curve and flatten. Repeat this palms up and then palms down sequence three more times.

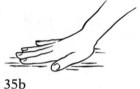

35a   35b

36   FINGER CIRCLES

STARTING POSITION: Hold your hands the same way you did for the Finger Fan (exercise 35).

THE EXERCISE: **(1)** Slowly circle your thumbs down, out, up, and back toward your second fingers. Take 8 counts to do this. **(2)** Now reverse the direction of the circle, starting up, out, down, and back toward your second fingers. Repeat these circles three more times. Now do these finger circles with each of your other fingers. Try to hold the nonworking fingers still and extended. This will be hard to do when you get to your ring and little fingers. Work at holding them still. Your finger muscles need this challenge. Repeat this entire sequence with your palms up. This new starting position changes which of your finger muscles is being stretched and which is being strengthened.

37   FINGER PRESSES

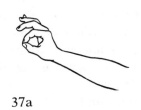

37a

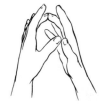

37b

STARTING POSITION: Hold your hands the same way you did for the Finger Fan (exercise 35).

THE EXERCISE: **(1)** Slowly press the tips of your thumbs and second fingers together, *37a*. Keep your knuckles round; don't let any of them become square. Press for 4 counts. **(2)** Relax your thumb and second finger. **(3)** Now press the tips of your thumbs and middle fingers together as you did for the second fingers. Press for 4 counts. **(4)** Relax your hand. **(5)** Now press the tips of your thumbs and ring fingers together. Press for 4 counts. **(6)** Relax your hand. **(7)** Press the tips of your thumbs and your little fingers together. Press for 4 counts. **(8)** Relax your hand. **(9)** Slowly extend your fingers out and apart to stretch them as wide and as far back as they will go.

Another way to do this exercise is to press the fingers of both your hands together so you won't overwork your thumbs. Hold the bottoms of your palms together and let the tips of your fingers touch, *37b*. Now firmly press your little fingers, then your ring fingers, and so forth in the same way as described above. {**Troubleshooting:** Be careful to prevent your knuckles from flattening or bending. Keep your fingers curved.}

38   SLOW PIANO PLAYING

This exercise is good for coordination, especially for the hand with which you do not write. That hand often is not as coordinated and needs attention. This exercise feels like slow piano playing of one note after the other with a regular slow rhythm. For each movement of your fingers, pretend that you are pushing your fingers through wet clay so that you give them a feeling of resistance. If you are a pianist, you won't need to do this exercise.

You will do this with your fingers extended and then with them curved.

STARTING POSITION: Hold your hands the same way you did for the Finger Fan (exercise 35).

THE EXERCISE: **(1)** With your palms down and fingers extended, press your thumbs down as though you were pushing into a piece of clay. Do this in 2 counts. Keep your thumbs there. **(2–5)** Now press your second fingers down. Do this in 2 counts. Keep them there. Continue pressing each finger in the same way, ending with your little finger. **(6–10)** Now you reverse the path that you just made with your fingers by first raising your little fingers, then your ring fingers, then your middle fingers, and so on. Do each of these movements in 2 counts. **(11)** Now turn your hands over so that your palms are facing up and repeat the sequence.

Now repeat this exercise with your fingers curved.

8 Your Rib Cage

Anatomy

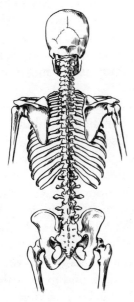

VIII-A

Your lungs and heart are housed in your rib cage *(VIII-A, VIII-B)*. It is shaped like a beehive with a triangular front opening. The floor of your rib cage is your diaphragm. This horizontally ribbed basket is very responsive to your breathing needs because of the way your ribs are attached in back to your bendable spine, and in front to cartilage that attaches to your sternum, or breastbone. This part of your spine, the thorax, is not as bendable as the cervical (neck) and lumbar (lower back) areas are. Your rib cage does have a range of movements. It expands, contracts, elevates, and relaxes, depending on your level of physical exertion, emotional response, or physiological need, such as sneezing or crying.

Your first rib is directly under your collarbone and is the smallest in circumference. Your next six ribs gradually enlarge in circumference but are similar to your first rib in their attachments to your spine in back and your sternum in front. Your next three ribs attach to your spine in back and to cartilage which then attaches to the bottom of your sternum. Your last two "floating" ribs attach to your spine but do not reach around to attach to any bone in front. Muscle attachments stabilize the front tips of these ribs.

Put your hands on your rib cage, first on the sides, then on

83

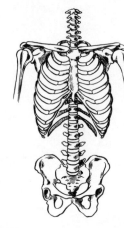

VIII-B

top under your collarbone, then in front and back, and take deep breaths. You can feel the range of motion of these bones. Now pretend to sneeze or force a cough and notice what your rib cage's responses are. Your ribs feel as though they expand because they lift and lower. Their cartilage attachments allow this movement to happen in the way that a bucket handle lifts and lowers on its attachment to the bucket. Each rib has this type of mobile attachment, and these joints are effectively held together by ligaments.

There are several layers of muscles in and around your rib cage. The floor of your rib cage, your diaphragm, is the major rib cage muscle. When this expands upward into your rib cage, it elevates your ribs and causes you to take an in-breath, to inhale. As your diaphragm relaxes, your ribs lower and you exhale. (Breathing is discussed further in Chapter 15.) You have three layers of muscle that vertically connect each rib along its entire surface to the rib below and above it. These layers essentially fill in the spaces between your ribs and hold them in line. You also have smaller and narrower muscles that reach diagonally from each rib to every other rib. These are located where your ribs join your spine and join your sternum. All these muscles cooperate during your breathing and enable your ribs to move in response to your other physical needs.

The muscles of your neck cooperate when you need to breathe very deeply. So do some of your shoulder blade muscles in back, some of your arm muscles in front of your chest, and your abdominal muscles below. They do this by remaining stationary, by holding still. This action is called stabilizing. These non–rib cage muscles assist your rib cage muscles to move in the greatest range necessary to get the job done. An example of this type of activity can be observed after a very fast race. Can you remember how much your chest heaves after you have exerted that much energy? Do you remember the feeling of holding your neck and arms still so that your ribs could expand fully? This cooperation of all your muscles happens automatically.

Except when you get a stitch in your side (see Chapter 16 for what to do), you probably don't pay much attention to your rib cage muscles. Keeping them mobile, stretched, and strong, however, is vital to your well-being. When you do aerobic activity, the kind of activity that promotes the supply and use of oxygen, you not only exercise your lungs, which breathe, and your heart, which efficiently circulates the oxygen, you also exercise your rib cage muscles. This stretching and strengthening benefits not just your rib cage, but also lessens the work of your abdominal and lower back muscles. Strengthening your rib cage muscles will benefit you more if you combine proper alignment with mobile and responsive muscles (see Chapter 15).

Exercises

39

CONE-SHAPED STRETCH

This stretch is good for getting the kinks out of your rib cage muscles so you can breathe deeply and freely. It is good to do before you begin any vigorous physical activity and after you have been sitting and concentrating over a desk or workbench.

STARTING POSITION: You can do this stretch either sitting or standing. If you are sitting, place your buttocks firmly against the back of your chair and press your feet on the floor, a foot or so apart. Hold in your abdominal muscles. If you are standing, place your feet apart about the distance of one of your own foot lengths. Another way to think about this distance is that your legs should come straight down from your hip sockets. Bend your knees a little in order to keep your lower back very vertical and thereby prevent any strain. Lift your arms up above your head. Extend them, but do not lock your elbows. Keep your shoulder blades down. Your arms are aligned with your ears.

THE STRETCH: **(1)** Reach your arms up as high as you can while still keeping your shoulder blades down. Try to touch the ceiling, *39a*. You should feel this stretch at the lower part of your rib cage in front and back. Hold that position until you feel the tightness in your muscles relax, about 10 to 15 counts. **(2)** Now reach sideways to the right toward the place in the room where the wall meets the ceiling, *39b*. You are reaching your arms on a high diagonal line. Do not curve at

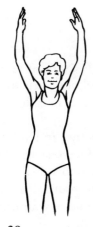

39a

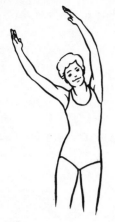

39b

the waist. You should feel this stretch along the left side of your ribs. Hold this position until you feel the tightness relax, about 10 to 15 counts. **(3)** To bring your rib cage upright again, specifically use the muscles on the left side of your rib cage to slowly lift your arms, neck, and head back up to your starting position. Take 4 slow counts to do this. (You can do this by just coming up, but that way simply uses momentum.) **(4)** Now reach sideways to the left in the same way as you did to the right. Hold this high diagonal position for 10 to 15 counts until you feel the tightness on the right side of your ribs relax. **(5)** Specifically use the muscles on the right side of your rib cage to slowly bring your upper body up to the first vertical position. Take 4 counts to do this. **(6)** Now pull your arms and ribs forward toward the place where the wall meets the ceiling. This is hard to do while keeping your shoulder blades down. Work to keep them held down. In order to do this part of this stretch, you need to keep your lower back vertical; don't let it tip forward at your hip sockets. The more firmly you hold in your abdominal muscles, the more you will feel this stretch in back along your rib cage. You are again pulling your arms and your upper body along a high diagonal. Hold this stretch until you feel these rib cage muscles relax, about 10 to 15 counts. **(7)** Now tell those back rib cage muscles to slowly pull your arms, neck, and head back up to your first vertical position. Now start again at step 1 and reverse the direction of your reaching, moving your rib cage, arms, and head to your left.

40   HIGH CHEST ARCH

The first part of the instructions for this exercise tells you how to learn the position and get the feel of it. It is difficult to do safely but important to learn in order to keep your spine mobile.

STARTING POSITION: The rib cage position in High Chest Arch is the same as in Floppy Push-ups (exercise 60). Sit on the floor tailor fashion, with your legs comfortably crossed. Feel that your weight is on and in front of your "sitz" bones. Hold on to your knees with your hands. Hold in your abdominal muscles, and align your back vertically.

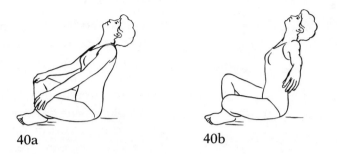

40a   40b

THE STRENGTHENING EXERCISE: Throughout the first part of this sequence of movements, be sure to hold on to your knees and monitor your lumbar vertebrae, the spine below your ribs. Do not allow it to arch back. **(1)** Tip your sternum (breastbone) back to try to make it parallel with the ceiling. This is not a big movement. Your rib cage will move only 3 to 4 inches back. As you learned in Chapter 4, you can tilt your head back while keeping your neck vertical; the next step requires that you do just that. **(2)** Now look up at the ceiling and make your face parallel with the ceiling, *40a.* {**Troubleshooting:** Do not drop your head back; hold your head with your front neck muscles and make sure you can talk. That is a test that you have not dropped your head back and partially closed your windpipe.} Once you have successfully put yourself in this position, then **(3)** bring up your arms and extend them sideways at shoulder level, *40b.* {**Troubleshooting:** If you start to fall over backward, straighten yourself back up, distribute your weight forward of your sitz bones, and begin again.} Hold this position for 5 to 10 counts, and then **(4)** bring your head up to a vertical position and bring your rib cage back up to a vertical position. Rest your arms down. Practice this sequence until you know the feel of the correct position. It is very important to keep your abdominals held firmly in and not to bend at the waist. When doing this exercise, be sure to pay attention to preventing pain in your lower back and keeping it vertical. *Sense* your body in front and back, and then this back diagonal position will be safe. You will feel mild stretching in the front lower part of your rib cage. Be careful not to feel any stretching in your abdominal muscles.

41

BACK RIB STRETCH

STARTING POSITION: This can be done standing, sitting in a chair or sitting tailor fashion on the floor. When standing, place your feet about 10 inches apart, relax your knees, hold in your abdominal muscles, and align your head so your ears are directly over your shoulders. When sitting in a chair, place your buttocks against the back of the chair and place your feet firmly on the floor close to the chair legs so that your feet can press down when you are doing the stretch. When sitting on the floor, sit tailor fashion so that your legs are comfortable. You may need to place something under your thighs to support them if your muscles are too tight to feel relaxed in this position.

THE STRETCH: (1) Tip your rib cage sideways a little to the right, about 3 inches from your vertical position. If you are sitting on the floor, extend your right arm to the floor and lean on your right hand to hold the tipped position. Now reach your left arm up, diagonally across your chest and out toward the place where the wall meets the ceiling, *41*. Actively pull that arm and at the same time pull down on your left hip. You should feel this stretch in the muscles in back below your ribs. {**Troubleshooting:** If you feel this stretch on the side of your rib cage, it is because you have twisted your rib cage to the right. Keep your rib cage facing front. When you are sitting, if you do not feel the stretch strongly in the back below your rib cage, it may be because you have tipped your torso forward on a diagonal and you need to keep it vertical. Only your arm should be diagonal.} Hold this stretch position 30 seconds to a minute. Now move your outstretched arm over to the left about 3 inches. When you do this, you should feel the stretch come closer to your spine in the back. Bring your arm down, and **(2)** repeat this stretch on the other side, leaning to your left and stretching your right arm diagonally across to your left. Remember to pull down on the right hip and to keep your rib cage forward and vertical. During the time you are doing this stretch, you can move your arm about 3 inches to the right to feel the stretch closer to your spine. This stretch is very helpful in relieving back pain.

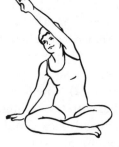

41

42

TORSO TURNS

In the next exercise you will move your rib cage, but the muscles that do the work are your abdominal muscles. Chapter 9 deals with the abdominal muscles, but this exercise is here because the area of the body you are *moving* is your rib cage. By learning to do Torso Turns, you can learn to move your upper body while keeping your lower back aligned. This habit can help protect your lower back from the mechanical stress that it experiences every day.

STARTING POSITION: You can do this exercise sitting or standing. To feel the way you will work with your muscles, try it first sitting and then do it standing. You can sit on the floor, *42a*, or on a chair. If you are sitting on a chair, sit forward so you will not bump into the chair back. Place your feet firmly on the floor about a foot apart. Hold in your abdominal muscles, and align your head so that your ears are directly over your shoulders. Let your arms hang down at your sides when you are learning the exercise. Then you can hold them extended out sideways at shoulder level or hold them extended over your head. When standing, place your feet apart so that your legs extend straight down from your hip sockets. Keep your knees unlocked and feel the entire surface of your feet pressing the floor. Align your upper body as described above.

THE STRENGTHENING EXERCISE: You will slowly turn your upper body around to the right. **(1)** First turn your rib cage, then **(2)** turn your neck, then **(3)** turn your head, and **(4)** look out the corner of your right eye and try to see something directly behind you. Keep your spine vertical. Take 2 counts to do each step. Make sure to keep your weight evenly distributed on both of your buttocks, *42b*. **(5)** Slowly bring

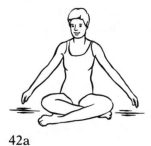

42a

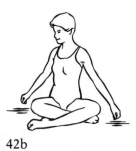

42b

your rib cage, neck, head, and eyes back to your beginning position. This part feels very easy, so be sure to move slowly, taking 8 counts. **(6)** Repeat the whole sequence to the left.

Turn to the right and left three more times each. Then try the sequence with your arms held out to your sides, and then with your arms extended above your head. When you do this exercise slowly, you can feel your waistline muscles working and they will become fatigued. {**Troubleshooting:** You may also feel discomfort in your lower back if you allow your pelvis to tilt forward. To prevent any lower back discomfort from this exercise, pay attention to any sensations you feel in your lower back. If you are doing this correctly, you should feel *no* sensation at all there.}

43   KNEE-CHEST POSITION

This position is useful for relieving menstrual cramps as well as for lessening the exaggerated curve that develops as a result of "round shoulder" posture.

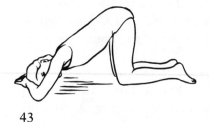

43

STARTING POSITION: Kneel on all fours on the floor or bed, with your hands directly under your shoulders. Feel that your thighs are straight up and not slanted back or forward. Hold in your abdominal muscles. *43.*

THE STRETCH: Bend your arms to rest yourself down on your forearms. Let your elbows point out, sideways, away from your body. Rest your head on the floor or bed, either on your forehead or on the side of your face. If you rest your head on its side, be sure to turn your head to rest on the other side after 30 seconds to a minute. You can rest in this position for 5 to 10 minutes. The correct position keeps your lumbar vertebrae straight. {**Troubleshooting:** Do not have any arch in your lower back. To prevent any arching, make sure that your arms are far enough forward before you bend your elbows to lower your chest to the floor.}

9   Your Abdominal Muscles

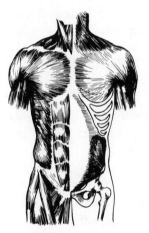

IX-A

Anatomy

Your abdominal muscles attach your rib cage to your pelvis, and thereby connect your upper body to your lower body *(IX-A)*. They also hold in your vital organs, and along with your spine in the back they help support your entire body in front. They really are responsible for a major part of your body's well-being, comfort, and mobility. And luckily, they respond to exercise more readily than any of the other muscles in your body.

This chapter is intimately connected to Chapter 10, "Your Lower Back and Hips," but because of their importance, your abdominal muscles have a chapter all to themselves. This is to emphasize how you can take care of them, strengthen them, and maintain their tone so they can do their job for you.

Unlike the other anatomical descriptions in this book, this one is entirely about muscles and not bones and ligaments. Like most of your body, your abdominal muscles are in layers. Like your neck muscles, these muscles cooperate on both sides of your body. Starting in front, you have a long vertical muscle running from the lowest part of your sternum to the top of your pubic bone, at the middle-front part of your pelvis. This muscle is the rectus abdominis. It is three to four inches wide. Underneath that is the linea alba ("white line"), which is a tendinous fibrous vertical unit to which your other abdominal muscles are attached. The external oblique attaches to the lower ribs and the linea alba in front, and reaches across your waist to attach to the top side of your pelvis in back. It runs on a diagonal from both sides toward the center like the letter *V*. The internal oblique is a diagonal muscle that runs underneath and in the opposite direction from the external oblique. These are your major abdominal muscles.

Underneath these is the transversalis abdominis, with horizontal fibers directly underneath your belly button and some diagonal fibers reaching down to your pubic bone. The transversalis attaches in back to a sheath of fiber, called fascia, which then attaches to your lumbar vertebrae. This muscle functions mainly to hold in your internal organs and assists with breathing. These are mainly in the category of automatic, reflex actions. In back you have the quadratus lumbaris, which attaches to your lumbar vertebrae and lowermost rib and reaches down to the top back edge of your pelvis. Since this muscle does not attach to your front abdominal muscles, it does not directly hold you together horizontally around your middle. It does help in vertical support and sideways motion in back.

You are very familiar with the range of movement of this area of your body. At rest, when you sit or stand, your abdominals relax and are passively stretching. You know that when you breathe, these muscles rise and fall when you are on your back, and go in and out when you are standing. When you lie on your back and lift your head and shoulders, your abdominal muscles contract. When you lift your knees toward your nose, your lower abdominals contract. However, when you stand, you need not use your abdominal muscles when you bend over because gravity pulls the weight of your head and chest forward without muscle action. You do use your abdominals when you are standing, sitting, or lying down, to twist your torso, your head, and chest to one side or the other.

The importance of these muscles centers on their role in protecting your lower back and specifically your disks from permanent injury. This idea will be made much clearer in

Chapter 10, "Your Back and Hips." In the meantime, try to develop an awareness of where your abdominal muscles are located in your body when you do the exercises to strengthen them.

Only mannequins have flat stomachs. Normal people like you and me have slightly or more than slightly protruding bellies. Because you breathe, your abdominal muscles move in and out, up and down. You can probably flatten your abdominal wall if you hold your breath, but you can't live very easily that way. Because your abdominal muscles are vertical when you stand and sit and therefore must hold in your "guts" while you go about your life, your tummy muscles tend to sag. Because you are preoccupied with all the other activities in your life, you do not pay constant attention to whether or not your abdominal muscles are held in. And because you may not have had correct posture training and adequate or correct exercises for your abdominal muscles, you are likely to have weak abdominals. Because these muscles are central in and central to your body and its well-being, the more faithfully, carefully, and correctly you strengthen them, the better off your body will be.

There are no exercises in this book to stretch your abdominal muscles. These muscles are always being mildly or severely stretched. The real challenge is to strengthen them adequately. The following exercises are the most effective ones available for strengthening these underworked muscles.

Exercises

44

ISOMETRIC ABDOMINAL STRENGTHENING

Any time you can think of doing this exercise, do it. Hold in your abdominal muscles. Hold for 8 to 10 counts. When you relax, take care not to let your muscles just fall forward. And pushing them out simply exaggerates the problem of overstretch that already exists. Relax them slowly.

45

PUSSY CAT

If you don't have enough strength in your abdominal muscles to gain benefit from curl-downs (exercises 47–49), then you need to start with Pussy Cat and Leg-Arm-Head Lifts (exercise 46). These are good exercises to do when you are recovering from an injured back. They are milder than regular curl-downs so you will have to repeat them more often to gain their strengthening benefits.

STARTING POSITION: Kneel on all fours on the floor, as though you were going to crawl. Make sure that your arms are straight down from your shoulders (do not lock your elbows) and that your thighs are straight down from your hip sockets. Rest the tops of your feet on the floor, straight back; don't let your feet toe in. The position of your body is like a table. Your back is flat and your arms and legs are like table legs, *45a*.

THE STRENGTHENING EXERCISE: (1) Tighten your abdominal muscles and let that action curve your back up into the shape of a hill or an upside-down bowl. You are hunching your back, *45b*. Do this action very slowly, taking 4 slow counts. It is possible to make your body move into this shape without using your abdominal muscles: you can just lift up your rib cage and tighten your buttocks to hunch your back. But the exercise is very effective if you use your abdominal muscles to do the job instead. **(2)** Slowly flatten out your back without untightening your abdominal muscles very much. Don't let your muscles relax or allow your back to arch, or make a concave curve. Take 4 slow counts to do this. Repeat this hunching up and flattening out of your back seven more times.

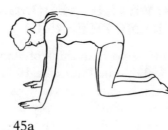

45a

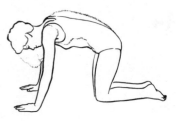

45b

46

LEG-ARM-HEAD LIFTS

STARTING POSITION: Lie on your right side. Bend your right leg so it gives you support and helps you stay on your side. Bend your right arm so you can rest your head on it like a pillow. Extend your left arm straight over your head, as though you were reaching for something on the floor above your head.

THE STRENGTHENING EXERCISE: **(1)** Lift your left leg up as far as it will go without turning your knee up to the ceiling. (Keep your knee forward.) Take 4 counts to do this and hold your leg there during steps 2–5, *46a.* **(2)** Now lift your extended left arm so that your arm is about 8 inches from your ear. Your arm is reaching on a diagonal and still above your head, *46b.* Take 4 counts to do this. **(3)** Now lift your head so that your left ear is moving toward your left shoulder, *46c.* Take 4 counts to do this. **(4)** Now lower your head back to rest on your bent right arm, taking 4 counts. **(5)** Lower your arm to the floor above your head, taking 4 counts. **(6)** Finally, lower your left leg to its starting position on the floor, taking 4 slow counts. Repeat the sequence of lifting your leg, then arm, then head, and lowering your head, arm, and leg seven more times. This exercise is to strengthen your side abdominal muscles, but it is milder than the side Curl-downs (exercise 47) so it has to be repeated more times. To make this more challenging, slow the counts down and use 6 counts to lift each part of your body and 6 counts to lower it. Continue to repeat the sequence eight times.

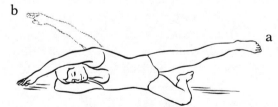

46

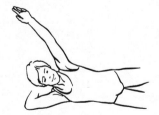

46c

47

CENTER

CURL-DOWNS

STARTING POSITION: Sit on the floor with your knees very bent, pointing up to the ceiling, and your feet 10 to 12 inches from your buttocks. Bring your chin in toward your neck and then curve your head forward so your chin is near your chest. When you actually do your curl-downs, you will cross your arms across your chest; but while you find the correct starting position, place your hands on your knees.

Now, here are three sitting positions that are not the correct ones in which to start curl-downs, but you must feel them in order to distinguish the correct starting position from the incorrect ones. Until you round your spine and transfer your upper body weight back far enough, the muscles called your hip flexors will be doing the work of lowering and lifting your upper body instead of your abdominal muscles, and thus you will not be strengthening the correct set of muscles.

The first incorrect position that you can feel is this first seated position, *47a*. You can feel your pointed "sitz" bones holding your weight on the floor. The second incorrect position is when you curve your spine and roll back a little, *47b*. There you will feel the fleshy part of your buttock muscles. Now roll back a little more and you will feel your coccyx, the small bone at the base of your spine, *47c*. This is very uncomfortable so curl yet farther back and down — and now, hurrah! You have arrived at the correct starting position, *47d*. Once you have found this position you can feel your topmost abdominal muscle begin to work. {**Troubleshooting:** Often this abdominal muscle will push out. Don't let this happen. If necessary, take an in-breath to pull in that muscle. When it pushes out, it is on "grab" stretch and that is exactly what you do *not* want.} Now place your arms across your chest, align your head, and keep your chin in as you did for the Center Neck Stretch (exercise 1), and begin the exercise.

THE STRENGTHENING EXERCISE: Before you begin, return to the first sitting position. Now — and this is very important — hold in your middle abdominal muscles, and again curl down to the correct starting position. Only now are you ready to begin the exercise. **(1)** Slowly roll back-

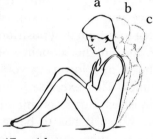

47   (three wrong starting positions)

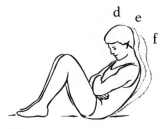

d e
   f

47

ward, down toward the floor, as though you could touch one vertebra at a time to the floor, *47d,e,f.* (In truth, you can't really do this because your spine is not quite that flexible.) As you lower your upper body backward, move your feet in toward your buttocks. This will keep your abdominal muscles doing the work and not your hip flexors. Roll down as far as you can and still remain in control. To the middle of your rib cage may be as far down as you will ever go when you develop enough strength to control this much uncurling. How far you uncurl depends on the strength of these muscles. At first you may only go a few inches before you need to start to curl up. That is fine. Tomorrow you will be able to uncurl an inch or so farther. If you uncurl too far, you will not be able to come up without a sudden toss or heave of your upper body, and then you are using momentum instead of strengthening your abdominal muscles. As you uncurl, keep your upper body rounded, your chin tucked in and on your chest, and keep your feet on the floor. At first, take 3 counts to uncurl, then as your muscles become stronger, take 4, then 5, then 6, 7, or 8. (Good luck if you consistently try 8!) **(2)** Reverse the path that your upper body just followed. Slowly curl up, keeping your body in the same rounded position. Pretend you are sitting inside a big tire. Initiate the curl-up at your forehead and that way you will keep your chin tucked in (and not strain your neck) and keep your arms relaxed on your chest (and not use them to help pull yourself up). Make sure to hold in your abdominal muscles! Curl up only to the correct starting position and not higher, otherwise you will have trouble getting comfortable when you start the side curl-downs. Take the same number of counts to curl up that you use to curl down. Keep your movement smooth and slow. Do not stop moving between the down and the up parts of this strenuous exercise. If you can't come up, you have uncurled too far. Only go down as far as you can control. As you gain strength, you will be able to uncurl farther down and control the change of direction.

Now you are ready to do the other two-thirds of a curl-down. You've only done one-third!

SIDE

STARTING POSITION: Side curl-downs need to have their starting position explained. It is important to remain in the correct starting position for the center curl-downs in order

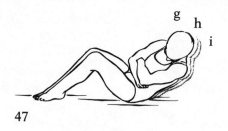

47

to get ready to do a side curl-down. In that correct rounded position, you now tip that entire shape to your left. That means that you are tipped sideways enough to have your right buttock off the floor. Now relax your head sideways over your left shoulder so that you can see the floor, *47g*. {**Troubleshooting:** If you feel a funny twing-twang under your left buttock, then you have come unrounded.} If you are in the correct position you will be resting on a triangle of your buttock that is comfortable to sit on during this part of the curl-down. **(3)** Uncurl your upper body inch by inch. Touch the side of your pelvis to the floor, then the side of your waistline, and then the lower back side of your rib cage, *47g,h,i*. Take 3 to 4 counts to do this — that is, only take the number of counts that you can control. **(4)** Curl up, staying in the same side position, with your right buttock off the floor. Keep your head relaxed and continue gazing down on the floor over your shoulder. This helps keep you from straining your neck and helps to keep you in the side position. Make sure to hold in your middle abdominal muscle. It may push out in a vain attempt to help your weak (because rarely used) side abdominal muscles. Keep your knees bent and your feet on the floor. **(5–6)** Tip your rounded body to the other side and repeat the side curl-down, following the instructions just given in steps 3 and 4.

You have just completed a single whole curl-down. You can see that it includes three positions: down and up in the center position, down and up to the left, and down and up to the right. Now you need to repeat this sequence two more times. The number of counts that you take for each part of the exercise will depend on your strength. Start at a count that your muscles can manage. Then increase the challenge as you become stronger. It is counterproductive to start with too many counts and not be able to bring your body up once you have gone down too far. So start with 3 or 4 counts down and use the same number of counts to come up. Use this count to each side, down and up. Use this count for a week. Then increase the count by one. Do the curl-down smoothly.

{**Troubleshooting:** Here are the most common mistakes or problems that you should avoid when you are doing curl-downs. Keep the middle muscle held in while doing the curl-down in all three positions. Don't let it push out at any time. If it does, either take an in-breath to pull it back in or come up a little until you can get it to come back in. Any time you are practicing it wrong is a waste of your time and teaches your muscles the wrong habit. On the side curl-downs, keep your head relaxed and looking down over your shoulder. Don't use it to help pull yourself up. Keep your feet moving toward your buttocks. Your legs will try to unfold and reach forward in an attempt to counterbalance the weight of your upper body falling, but such leg action will prevent your abdominal muscles from doing the work. Keep your body curved or rounded all the time. When doing the side curl-downs, make sure to keep your weight on one buttock during the entire time you are doing both the down and up parts of the exercise.}

48   COMPROMISE CURL-DOWNS

If you find Pussy Cat and Leg-Arm-Head Lifts (exercises 45, 46) too easy and regular Curl-downs (exercise 47) too hard, here is what to do to bridge the gap between the two exercises.

STARTING POSITION: Put your hands on your knees and then lower yourself into the lowest position of a correct center curl-down. Make sure to hold in your rectus abdominis muscle.

THE STRENGTHENING EXERCISE: **(1)** Let go of your knees, keep your arms extended just above your knees, *48*, and see if you can hold the correct position for 4 to 6 counts. **(2)** Hold on to your knees again and curl your rib cage up about 2 inches. Take your hands away again and hold that position for 4 to 6 counts. **(3 and 4)** Repeat this process, coming up 2 inches at a time until you are in the correct starting position for regular curl-downs. Once you can do this with

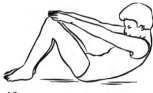

48

relative ease, then cross your arms on your chest each time you let go of your knees. This arm position is more difficult because when your arms are extended forward, they help to cantilever your lower body. When you cross your arms on your chest, your abdominal muscles must hold up more weight.

49   WALL CURL-DOWNS

These curl-downs are much harder to do than the regular curl-downs because they make it even more certain that your hip flexors will not help your abdominal muscles.

STARTING POSITION: Sit near a wall so you can put your feet up on it at a right angle to your thighs. Position yourself so that your weight is on the same starting place as for regular curl-downs, *49a*. You are not on your sitz bones or your coccyx, but you are on the lower part of your spine. Don't put your entire foot on the wall. That will make it too easy for you to push against the wall when you are lowering and raising your upper body. Extend your ankles and rest your toes lightly against the wall, but at no time during the down and up should you push them against the wall. Cross your arms on your chest, tuck in your chin, and keep your neck rounded forward.

THE STRENGTHENING EXERCISE: **(1)** Uncurl your upper body down as far as you can control the lowering without letting your middle abdominal muscle push out, *49a, b, c.* Take 3 to 4 counts to do this. **(2)** Slowly curl back up to your correct starting position. **(3)** Tip your entire body to the left and make sure that your right buttock is off the floor, *49d.*

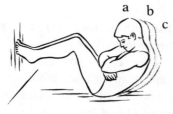

49

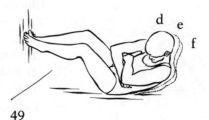

49

Relax your head over your left shoulder and see the floor below that shoulder. Now uncurl down toward your waist and then toward your ribs. Take 3 to 4 counts. When you feel you cannot control your lowering body, *49d,e,f,* **(4)** curl back up, keeping your body rounded, your right buttock off the floor, and your head relaxedly hanging over your left shoulder. **(5–6)** Repeat this sequence on the right. Repeat the down-and-up sequence in the middle, and to each side two more times. Take the same precautions as in regular curl-downs.

10 Your Lower Back and Hips

Anatomy

Two parts of your spine have already been described in the chapters on your neck and your rib cage. This chapter is about your lower back (the lumbar area of your spine) and your hips (the common name of your pelvic girdle). The base of your spine, your sacrum and coccyx, are tightly joined in the back of your pelvis. Because your spinal column sits in and on your pelvis, these parts of your body coordinate in movements of either part. Before telling you about your lower back and hips, a description of the structure of your spine will help you understand how to protect it *(X-A, X-B, X-C)*.

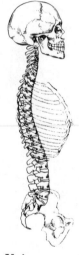

X-A

SPINE

Dr. Paul C. Williams has described the spine as a pile of hockey pucks and jelly donuts. In many ways, this metaphor can help you visualize the shape and texture of the parts of your spine. The weight-bearing part of each vertebra is lozenge shaped, like a hockey puck. The rest of each bone that attaches to this lozenge looks like three points of a star. The

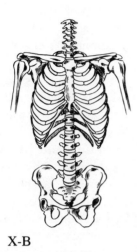

X-B

front view

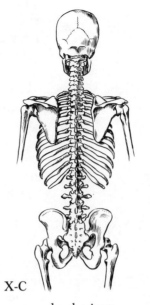

X-C

back view

direction in which the points of these bones protrude depends upon their location in your neck, your rib cage, or your lower back. The bumps that you can feel on your back are the bones that point diagonally down in your neck; vertically in your rib cage; and horizontally in your lower back. These varied shapes allow or prevent the kind of movement that each part of your spine can or cannot do. The parts of each vertebra are fused together. The protruding parts of each bone are also connected by ligaments and many little muscles, which allow some and prevent other types of movement, depending on which part of your spine they are in.

The stack of hockey pucks (the round part of your vertebrae) and the jelly donuts (the intervertebral disks) make up the weight-bearing part of your spine, and this special structure also allows for your spine's unusual mobility. The disks work like hydraulic shock absorbers. The center of each disk contains a thick fluid that absorbs shocks to your spine, such as jumping causes, and allows your spine to bend and twist in the many ways it does. The problem with your disks is that they degenerate, and as they do, some of their fluid

103

leaks out. With acute damage, some of the fluid can suddenly pop out. This can happen if you repeatedly move in ways that are unsafe for your spine. The case of each disk has few pain sensory nerve endings, so you cannot tell when you are hurting it until the damage you do is permanent. Sad to say, your disks won't regenerate the way the rest of your body's tissues do. Instead, fibrous tissue, like the calluses you get on the bottoms of your feet, replaces the fluid, so your disk is harder and narrower than it was and does not cushion your bones as before.

Damage to disks occurs most frequently in the lower back and next most frequently in the neck. The risks of damage are greatest in these areas because of the shape of those specific vertebrae and their resulting range of motion. Even if your spine can move forward and back with great freedom at your neck and in your lower back, this does not mean it is a good idea to do extreme movements. Back bends in gymnastics or head rolls found in common warm-up exercise sequences can cause permanent damage to your disks.

LOWER BACK

You have a wide range of motion in your lower back: forward in flexion; back in extension; even farther back into hyperextension or back arching; sideways in lateral flexion; and around in rotation. Your lumbar vertebrae have limited rotation. The reason that you can turn and look behind your back when you are sitting is that your neck and rib cage areas are able to rotate.

When you rotate your spine, the shape of your lumbar disks is such that your vertebrae slide sideways a little. And when your spine moves sideways, your lumbar vertebrae rotate a little. This causes a small amount of stress on the disks, ligaments, and muscles of the lumbar area, so you should be aware that these movements cause extra wear on this part of your spine. This stress is the least severe when your spine is vertical. The more you bend sideways and turn, the greater the stress on your spine. There are no side bending exercises in this book for that reason and the exercises that use rotation keep your body in a vertical position to protect your spine.

You have lots of muscles in your back, but none of them are very long or very strong. The muscles that you can massage on either side of your spine are part of a group that reaches up your spine in three steps: to the top of the lumbar area, to the middle of your rib cage, and to the middle of your neck. There are short muscles that connect the pointed parts of each of your vertebrae to each other and to your ribs in your thoracic spine. These muscles help your spine bend, extend, rotate, and move to each side. As you know, your abdominal muscles also contribute to the support and movements of your spine. By this time, you are probably becoming very aware of how highly coordinated the parts of your body are with each other.

PELVIS

Besides being your center of gravity, your pelvis plays a central role in supporting and moving your body. Your spine connects to the top back of it (with the fused part of your spine and tail bone going straight through it) and your legs attach to the bottom sides of it. So this bone supports your upper body when you sit, stand, or walk, and it carries and balances your body on your legs when you move, as in walking, running, and jumping. It has a curved, basinlike shape. Each of your hip bones is made up of three bones, which fuse during puberty. Your pubic bones are joined together in front by a thick disk of cartilage. The fused part of your spine, your sacrum and coccyx, are attached in the back middle of your hip bones. On each side are deep cup-shaped sockets for your thigh bones' ball-shaped ends to fit into. These bones are tightly connected with ligaments. The ligaments of your thigh bone are structured freely enough to allow your legs their wide range of motion.

The movement of your pelvis depends on what your spine or legs are doing. You can move it front, back, to each side, and around. Do each of these movements while you are sitting and feel how the lumbar area of your spine moves along with your pelvis. Now do these movements standing. If you don't bend your knees, you won't be able to move your pelvis very much at all. Because your pelvis coordinates with your spine and thighs, there are no muscles just for your pelvis. The muscles that control its movement are either of your spine or legs. And your abdominal muscles, which attach in front, are always part of this action, either passively or actively.

One of the major hip flexors, your psoas (pronounced "só-us") attaches to the sides of the lumbar vertebrae, passes inside the pelvis, and attaches to the top of the thigh bone, just below its socket *(X-D)*. This muscle can be responsible for low-back pain if you do not stand correctly aligned (Chapter 16). It is often very tight and needs stretching. Several of the lower back stretches in this chapter help relieve the tightness in this muscle. If you hold in your abdominal muscles to stabilize your pelvis, your psoas muscle can powerfully assist your thigh to move forward, to flex. You have another hip flexor inside your pelvis that works with your psoas.

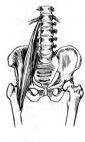

X-D

The shape of your buttocks is determined by the muscles that attach the thigh to the pelvis and help to move it *(X-E)*. Remember, you can't move your thigh when walking without moving your pelvis or, when stationary, without using the muscles attached to your pelvis. The muscles in your buttocks move your thigh sideways (away from your body) and backward. You use these same muscles when you stand up after bending forward, because they assist in bringing the back of your pelvis into a vertical position. Other muscles that move your pelvis are the quadriceps group of thigh muscles on the front of your thighs, your hamstrings in the backs of your thighs, and your inner-thigh muscles, which bring your legs back in toward your midline after they have been lifted out to the side. These thigh muscles and your gluteal muscles cooperate to rotate your thighs in and out. This cooperation is most needed when you walk because as you transfer your weight from one foot to another, all of your body weight is balanced for a moment on one leg and then the other. Your pelvic muscles adjust your entire body weight over each leg with every step you take.

Though it is possible to strengthen your buttock muscles,

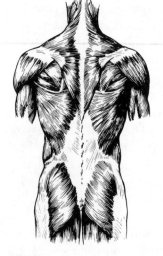

X-E

it is very difficult to strengthen your lower back. The exercises for strengthening your abdominal muscles and the downward depressors of your shoulder blades can help strengthen the area, but because of your back's structure, there are very few safe ways to strengthen the muscles of your entire back. You have muscle groups that serve each part of your spine but no large ones that are postural, that is, that really support your entire back. Chicken (exercise 15) in Chapter 5, with the leg extensions, is a safe and effective exercise to strengthen your entire back. It is an adapted version of an orthopedic corrective exercise. The muscles in your lower back, however, are usually too tight, too contracted, because of poor posture, weak abdominal muscles, and poor walking habits. The stretching positions in this chapter help you pull out tightness in your lower back. You can use all of them every day or only when you feel lower back pain.

The other major way for you to care for your lower back is to keep your calf and hamstring muscles stretched: see Chapters 11 and 12. The section on Alignment (exercise 98) in Chapter 15 explains why these stretches are so important to protect your lower back, and Chapter 16 explains what to do about many common back problems.

Exercises

50   DOOR FRAME PULL

This stretch is good to do if you have a backache or spasm in your lower back.

STARTING POSITION: Stand in a door frame with your toes about 12 inches back from the floor line of it. Hold on to the door frame at about shoulder height and extend your arms so you lean back slightly. Grasp the door frame with your thumbs down so your fingers wrap the frame and will be able to hold your weight when you pull back. Bend your knees as though you were about to sit down. Keep your rib cage and your pelvis vertical, one directly above the other.

107

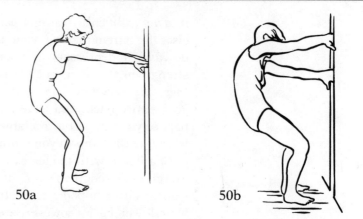

50a   50b

THE STRETCH: Pretend someone punched you in the stomach, *50a.* Or pretend that a big beach ball was pushed into your torso. The stretch happens when you simply pull back from the door frame and tuck your buttocks under a little. You feel the stretch in the place where lower back pain is so often experienced, the area down the spine inside your pelvis where you can't massage but have always wanted to. Hold this position as long as necessary to release the tightness in your back.

You can stretch one side and then the other in two ways. Place your right hand on the door frame about 6 inches higher than shoulder height, and then tilt your head to the left and move your pelvis a little to your right, *50b.* You should now feel the stretch on the right side of your lower back more than on the left. To feel it on your left side, put your right hand down where it was and place your left hand on the door frame 6 inches higher than shoulder height. Tilt your head to the right and move your pelvis a little to the left.

The other way to feel the stretch on each side separately is to assume the original starting position and just curve your torso to the right or to the left. Think banana shape for your rib cage, waist, shoulder, and head. At the same time as you curve sideways, also keep pulling back from the door frame and tucking under your buttocks. {**Troubleshooting:** You need to keep your rib cage over your pelvis. If you only pull back with your buttocks, you will not feel the stretch in your lower back.}

This stretch can be done with another person instead of a door frame. The person preferably should be your height and weight, but you can balance with almost anyone, with a little adjustment. Stand less than both of your arms' length apart, grasp each other's hands, and lean back so your arms are extended and you are keeping each other from falling. Now bend your knees and pretend to get punched in the stomach. Tuck your buttocks under a little and let your lower back pull back. The feeling of stretch in this position is the same as that of the Door Frame Pull. You can stretch each side by just raising your right and your partner's left arm about 6 inches. You will need less side adjustment of your pelvis and head to feel the side stretches. Repeat this on the other side, your left and your partner's right. Hold this stretch as long as necessary to release the tightness in your back.

51

SUPER BACK REST

This is a resting position more than an exercise. It is here because it is one of the most restful positions, especially if you have lower back pain.

RESTING POSITION: You need to have a chair, bed, sofa, or foot stool that is as high as your thighs are long. Lie down on the floor and put your lower legs up on this raised and comfortable surface so that your legs are fully supported, *51*. The surface must allow you to put your thighs beyond a right angle (i.e., nearer your chest). If you are resting your legs on a chair, you need to slide your buttocks under the chair just a little so your knees are pointing toward you.

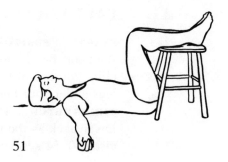

51

Then relax your arms out to your sides or down at your sides. Relax your jaw and lengthen your neck so it is not arched. After resting in this position for about 30 seconds, the area in your lower back that arches may hurt a little more than it did after 5 or 10 seconds. That stronger sensation is in the muscles that are tight as they begin to stretch out. That sensation should diminish markedly and soon you should have little or no pain sensation in that area. For more comfort, place a small rolled-up towel under your buttocks just below your tail bone. This should help keep your pelvis in such a position that your lower back will remain relaxed. Rest in this position for 5 to 10 minutes if you have time. Even 2 to 5 minutes will help relieve your back pain a lot.

You can sleep in this position on the floor if you put a foam pad under your back, or better yet, put the sofa cushions on your bed so your resting surface is comfortable. Support your head on either side with small pillows, but don't put a pillow under your head unless you really need it, and then it should be no more than about an inch thick.

Sometimes resting in this position for only 10 minutes can relax a sore lower back enough to allow you to get up and go about your daily business with much less pain. You can rest like this as often as you need to. It provides the same stretching in a horizontal position as the Door Frame Pull (exercise 50) provides you in a vertical position. {**Trouble-shooting:** If you feel pressure on your spine bones, make sure to lie on something soft. Place support on each side of your spine, such as towels folded lengthwise. This should relieve any bone pressure and let your muscles relax.}

52   PAUL WILLIAMS'S BACK STRETCH

STARTING POSITION: Lie on your back on your bed or on the floor. Bend your knees and bring them up toward your chin. You are in the fetal position on your back. Hug your legs under your knees or hold the tops of your knees.

THE STRETCH: This stretch relaxes the same area of your lower back as the two stretches just described above (exercises 50, 51). In order to feel this area of your lower back

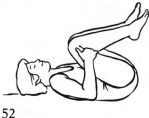

52

stretch, you need to pull your thighs close enough to your chest so that you pick up the lower part of your buttocks, *52*. Hold this position for 30 seconds to a minute, or until you feel the tightness in your lower back relax. Hold in your abdominal muscles. {**Troubleshooting:** Don't make the mistake of just squeezing your thighs against your chest and not lifting your tailbone. That won't really stretch out the tight area in your lower back. It may stretch your hamstrings (the muscle group on the back of your thighs) a little, but there are more effective stretches for these muscles. Hamstring stretches are described in Chapter 11.}

If this stretch is uncomfortable, then simply rest your bent legs toward your chest with your knees angled toward your armpits. Use your hands to lightly hold them in place.

53

CHIROPRACTIC POSITION

This is another way to relieve pain and tightness in your lower back.

STARTING POSITION: Lie on your back. Relax your jaw and your neck so it is not arched. Rest your arms out to your sides at shoulder height. Extend your right leg on the floor. Bend your left leg and bring your knee up so your left foot is very close to your buttocks.

THE STRETCH: Cross your bent left leg over your right, *53a*. Place your right hand on the top of your left thigh near your knee and pull your knee down toward the floor, *53b*. The angle at which you are pulling your leg down to the floor is not a right angle. You should pull your leg down to

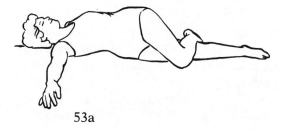

53a

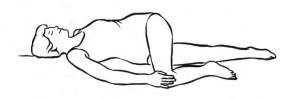

53b

the floor toward your foot, on a low diagonal. Keep your left shoulder close to the floor. Let your extended right leg roll over, but try to keep both of your shoulders on the floor. You will feel the stretch on the left side of your lower back and along the top of your buttocks muscles. Hold this position for 30 seconds to a minute. Repeat it on the other side. You are likely to feel this stretch on one side of your body more than the other because back pain usually is on one side more than the other. Hold the stretch as long as you need to, on the side that is tighter. You might feel it more completely if you start by putting your crossed-over knee on the floor and then pull your left shoulder back down toward the floor. Doing the stretch this way starts the pull from your upper body, whereas the other way starts the stretch from your leg, your lower body.

If the starting position on your back is difficult for you, you can accomplish the same thing starting from a side-lying position. Lie on your right side with your right arm out from under you. Bend your left leg so your left foot lies on your right knee or calf, and the left knee touches or almost touches the floor. Put your right hand on the left knee so you can give it some weight to hold it near the floor. Bring your left arm back to lie on the floor behind you, and let your shoulder girdle, neck, and head follow it back so the top half of your body is almost flat on the floor while the lower half twists to put the left knee down on your right side. Feel the stretch along the lower part of your left back and through the left buttock. Repeat to the other side.

54

OPEN TAILOR SIT

If when you try this stretch you feel discomfort on top of your thighs near your hip sockets, then you need to do the Sitting Quadriceps Stretch and Deep Lunge (exercises 61, 66) in Chapter 11 before you will be able to feel this stretch in your buttocks. This discomfort is common for those of you who have loose ligaments.

STARTING POSITION: Sit on the floor, tailor fashion, with your legs crossed in front of you, but instead of resting one

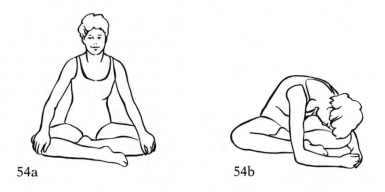

54a   54b

of your legs on top of your feet, move your legs apart a little and your front foot forward a little, so that your legs are not resting on your feet. Your legs are still placed in the same shape that they are in when you sit tailor fashion, *54a*.

THE STRETCH: Bend your upper body forward over the foot that is in front of your legs, *54b*. That is, if your right foot is in front of your left, then bend over diagonally to the left in the direction that your right toes are pointing. Your upper body will be bent over your right foot and your left knee. Keep your body over your foot and inside your knee. Let your head relax and hang down. Place your bent arms in front of your legs and on the floor. You will feel this stretch in your right buttocks muscles, very near your spine and tailbone. When you repeat this stretch on the other side, you need to put your left foot in front of your right and bend your upper body diagonally right over your left foot and inside your right knee. {**Troubleshooting:** If you feel some discomfort in your hip sockets, adjust your legs by moving your thighs a little closer together, opening them wider apart sideways, or separating them so that your front leg is more forward. Move your legs around to see if you can avoid this discomfort. Remember, you may need to stretch the muscles on the top of your thighs.} This stretch pulls out the tightness in the buttocks that results from what people call "sciatica" (see Chapter 16).

55

HALF PRETZEL

The Half Pretzel and the Pretzel (exercise 56) stretch the muscles on the sides of your buttocks and the top sides of your thighs. This area is not often stretched, so when you try it for the first time you may feel the stretching sensation very strongly. Hold the position as long as you can, because stretching these muscles enables your legs to move more freely back as well as forward. The Pretzel stretches also help relieve some of the discomfort that comes from low-back pain. When you are in pain your muscles tighten, and often this tightness has no natural way of relaxing or being pulled out.

Do the milder Half Pretzel if your muscles are very tight, or if the Pretzel gives you any discomfort in your knees. Eventually you will be able to do the whole Pretzel. Before you do either the Half Pretzel or the Pretzel, always stretch your quadriceps (exercise 61).

STARTING POSITION: Sit on the floor with your legs crossed tailor fashion. At first, move the leg that is in front — say it is your right leg — forward a little so you can put your left leg in the correct starting position. Move your left leg, which is bent on the floor, so that your knee is directly out in front of your midline, in front of your belly button, *55a*. Your left foot is near your right buttock. Don't sit on that foot. Now cross your right foot over your bent left leg and put your foot facing straight ahead on the floor on the left side of your left thigh, as though you were going to step on that foot.

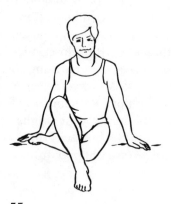 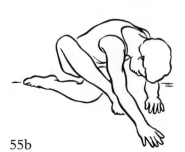

55a   55b

THE STRETCH: Bend your upper body sideways to the left so that you are resting your weight on your left forearm on the floor. Relax your head forward and put your right arm forward on the floor. Now press your right buttock toward the floor, *55b*.

You should feel the stretch on the side of your right thigh and in the buttock muscles directly above that area. Move your left arm forward as your buttock sinks to the floor. Keep your head relaxed forward. As you move your upper body more and more forward, your right leg will automatically change position. Your foot will come off the floor. Let this happen! Hold this position for 30 seconds to a minute.

Repeat the Half Pretzel on the other side. Place your right leg bent on the floor, with its knee in front of your belly button and your left foot on the floor on the right side of your right thigh. Lean your upper body to the right and rest your weight down on your right forearm. Notice if you are tighter on one side than the other. Hold the stretch position longer on your tighter side.

56

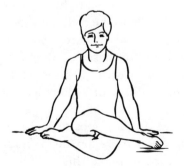

56a

PRETZEL

Always stretch your quadriceps (61, 62, 63, 64, or 65) and do Half Pretzel before you do Pretzel.

STARTING POSITION: Your underneath leg position is the same as for Half Pretzel (exercise 56). It is very important that you put the leg that is resting on the floor in the correct position, because otherwise you may feel discomfort in your knee or hip socket. Make sure that your left knee (and then your right) is directly in front of your midline, in front of your belly button. Now cross your right leg on top of your left so that your right knee is as much on top of your left as you can put it, *56a*. Your right foot is diagonally back toward your left hip. Flex that foot; that is, bend your ankle so that it is at a right angle to your lower leg. Your goal is to place your legs, one on top of another, so that they are the same shape, like the letter *V* but with your feet sticking out on each side. {**Troubleshooting:** When your knees are as much on top of each other as possible, then you should feel no discomfort in your knees. If you have discomfort in your

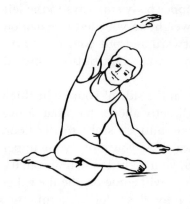

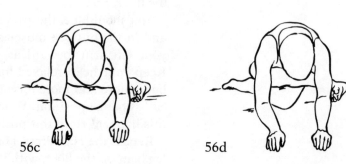

56b   56c   56d

hip sockets, place a 2–4-inch support, pillow or phone book, under your lower knee. See Troubleshooting at the end of 56.}

THE STRETCH: **(1)** Bend your upper body to your right and rest your weight on your right hand (or your right forearm if your muscles are flexible enough to do this), *56b*. Hold this position for 30 seconds. **(2)** Now bend your upper body to your left and rest your weight on your left hand or left forearm. Hold this position for 30 seconds, or until you feel the tightness lessen. **(3)** Now bend your upper body forward and move your arms forward in front of your legs on the floor, *56c*. Relax your head and let it hang down over your knees. You should feel this stretch on both sides of your thighs and the sides of your buttocks. Hold this position for 30 seconds to a minute, or as long as it takes to feel these tight muscles relax. **(4)** Move your upper body a little to the right and then to the left so you are on a slight diagonal forward, *56d*. You may feel the stretch more completely in these two diagonal positions rather than in the straight forward position. Hold these positions for 30 seconds to a minute or as long as you feel you need to hold.

Repeat this stretch with your legs in the opposite position. When this area of your body becomes more flexible as a result of stretching it, you may want to make this stretch a little stronger. The way to make the stretch stronger is to bend forward at your hip sockets. Above, you were instructed to bend your upper body forward. That usually happens at your waist and you bend forward from your rib cage. By bending forward from your hip sockets, the stretch will be stronger and you will protect your lower back from the slight discomfort that some people experience in the Pretzel. {**Troubleshooting:** Always remember to hold in your abdominal muscles. If you have any low-back discomfort after these suggestions, then instead of letting your head relax forward, keep your head and neck straight in line with your spine and hold in your chin. And gently hold in your abdominal muscles. These slight adjustments should prevent any low-back discomfort. Also, remember to do Half Pretzels if you need to work up to the full Pretzel.}

57   KEGEL EXERCISE

During the next two exercises, the Hip Curl and Jumping in Your Chair (exercises 58, 59), women can take the opportunity to tighten the muscles on the vaginal floor. This is known as the Kegel exercise, named for Dr. Arnold Kegel. You can do this exercise any time you think of it. And men can slowly and gradually tighten the muscles on the pelvic floor during exercises 58 and 59.

58   HIP CURL

This exercise is often called the "pelvic tilt." This version of it enables you to feel the muscles that you need to use to accomplish the movement. It also feels good to do if you have low-back pain. It can be done in bed as well as on the floor. Also, don't forget to tighten your pelvic floor (exercise 57).

STARTING POSITION: Lie on your back on the floor or bed. Bend your knees and put your feet very near your buttocks, *58a*. Relax your jaw and lengthen your neck so it is not arched. Place your arms out to your sides at shoulder height. As you do this exercise, press your toes so that you distribute your weight evenly on your feet. This will prevent your hamstrings from cramping.

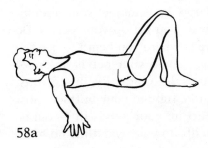

58a

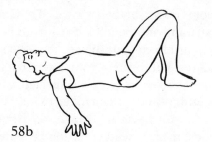

58b

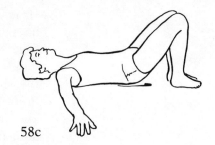

58c

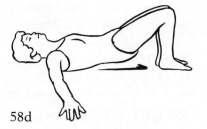

58d

THE STRENGTHENING EXERCISE: This is a cumulative series of small movements. **(1)** Tighten your buttock muscles as though you were going to tuck your pelvis under, but don't lift your pelvis. Just tighten the muscles. This tightening is along the bottom of your buttocks, not squeezing the buttocks together. As you tighten these buttock muscles, you should also feel in the front of your body that your abdominal muscles flatten toward the floor, *58b.* Take 4 counts to accomplish the tightening. **(2)** Now relax your muscles in 4 counts. As you relax these muscles, don't let your lower back come off the floor, *58a.* **(3)** Repeat step 1, tightening your buttocks, *58b,* and abdominal muscles, so that you just begin to curl up your pelvis, but not your waistline, *58c.* This movement is not very large. You can feel your abdominal area become even flatter as you lift up your pelvis. Do this in 4 counts, 8 in all. Here is where you begin to need to press your toes. **(4)** Now press down your pelvis, taking 4 counts. Relax your buttock muscles gradually, in 4 counts. **(5)** Repeat steps 1 and 3: that is, tighten your buttock muscles in 4 counts, *58b,* then curl up your pelvis in 4 counts, and now curl a bit farther to lift up your waistline no more than an inch off the floor, in 4 counts, 12 in all. **(6)** Reverse this slow curling pathway by unrolling and pressing down your spine piece by piece, taking 4 counts; your pelvis in 4 counts; and relaxing your buttock muscles in 4 counts. **(7)** Repeat steps 1, 3, and 5, *58b,c.* Now add a slight further curl by lifting up your lower two or three ribs, *58d.* Keep pressing your toes. Keep your abdominal muscles held in. Take 4 counts for each part, 16 counts in all. **(8)** Reverse this sequence by lowering your ribs in 4 counts, then your waistline in 4 counts. (This is actually impossible to do, because your spine is not quite flexible enough, but trying to do this works the muscles around the area in a beneficial way.) Then lower your pelvis in 4 counts, and relax your buttock muscles in 4 counts. You can repeat this sequence from the beginning or just repeat the last two parts, steps 7 and 8, three more times.

With the addition of a variety of leg movements, this final Hip Curl position is good to use to strengthen your inner and outer thigh muscles. A description of that part of the exercise is in Chapter 12.

59   JUMPING IN YOUR CHAIR

The buttock muscles that you just used to start the Hip Curl (exercise 58) are the same muscles that you automatically use when you start to jump. You can strengthen these muscles any time you feel like doing so when you are sitting in a chair or on the floor. Just tighten your buttock muscles. You will feel them tighten by squeezing together and starting to tuck under. Experiment with each of these actions. **(1)** Tighten in 4 counts. While you do this, take the opportunity to tighten your abdominal muscles also. As usual, doing this slowly, in 4 counts, is beneficial. **(2)** Slowly relax your muscles in 4 counts. Repeat this sequence three more times. Then do it faster, using 2 counts to contract your muscles and 2 counts to relax. Repeat this sequence three more times. While you do this exercise, also tighten your pelvic floor (exercise 57).

60

FLOPPY PUSH-UPS

Robin McKenzie, a physical therapist from New Zealand, has been teaching the use of Floppy Push-ups as a means of easing the back pain that comes from too much forward rounding of the lumbar area of the spine. Many people have had the awful experience of bending over to pick up something and not being able to come back up. You can do the High Chest Arch (exercise 40) or Floppy Push-ups to get immediate relief from that kind of pain. Slouched sitting can cause the same kind of back pain. Floppy Push-ups gently stretch the back muscles at the top of the lumbar area of the spine and bottom of the rib cage.

STARTING POSITION: Lie on your stomach with a small pillow across your middle between your hip bones and your ribs. The pillow supports your lower back. When you lie on your stomach, your lower back sags and arches because your rib cage is usually not the same circumference as your hip bone and so it sticks out farther. Put your hands under your shoulders, extend your head directly forward, and keep your chin in. Rest the tops of your feet flat on the floor or bed; that is, untuck your toes, *60a*.

THE EXERCISE: Slowly push your chest up about 8 to 10 inches by starting to straighten your elbows, *60b*. Take 4 counts to do this. Hold this position for 4 counts. Slowly lower your chest to the floor, *60a*. You will bend your spine at the junction of your rib cage and lower back. Repeat this several times and if comfortable hold for 6 to 8 counts. {**Troubleshooting:** If this hurts your back, don't do it. It is inappropriate for anyone with a degenerated disk to do this exercise; so if it hurts, stop!} This exercise is helpful for those of you with a lumbar area that does not bend back very easily, because a spine that is too straight can be just as problematic as one that is too severely curved.

60

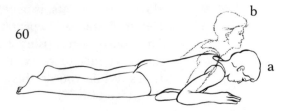

11 Your Thighs: Front and Back

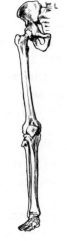

XI-A

Anatomy

You know from reading the anatomy section of Chapter 10, "Your Lower Back and Hips," that your thigh muscles are attached to your pelvis and that they help move your pelvis. Now it's time to think about your thighs and their next attachment, in your knee joint *(XI-A)*.

Your thigh bone, the femur, starts in your hip socket and ends at your knee. It is one long, solid, slightly bowed bone. At your pelvis, it has a ball-shaped end, which fits deeply into your hip socket. At your knee, it has two flattened ball-shaped bumps side by side, with a groove in between them. This end fits into the protruding triangular eminence of the tibia, the stronger of your two lower leg bones. The fibula, your other lower leg bone, attaches to the side of the tibia. At the top end of your tibia is a half-moon-shaped cartilage that makes a deeper socket for your femur to bend and straighten in. Your knee joint is held together with vertical ligaments on the sides; with two crossing ligaments from the bottom of the femur to the top of the tibia; with a ligament that also holds the patella, or kneecap, in place; and with the tendons of some of your thigh and calf muscles. Your knee is constructed for mobility and is surrounded by some of your strongest muscles. It is also structured to provide stability to your entire body. But because of the work it does, your knee is very vulnerable. It is the most injured part of the body in sports and dance, so special care must be taken to use it correctly.

You thigh moves forward and back and from side to side, and a combination of these directions allows you to move it in big circles. You can move your thigh in these directions whether your lower leg is straightened or bent. Your lower leg bends and extends at your knee. Standing is the only function your lower leg is meant to perform. When you do not have weight on your lower leg and your knee is bent, you can turn your foot in and out. Part of this movement happens in your ankle but a lot of it happens at your knee. These rotary motions are meant to occur when you are *not* bearing weight on your knee. If you are bearing weight and your movement twists your knee, that is when and how you can injure it.

Most of your thigh muscles have two jobs. They move your thigh in its many directions and also bend and extend your lower leg at your knee. (In Chapter 13, "Your Lower Leg," you will learn more about the muscles that reach from your thigh to your lower leg.) In the front of your thighs are your four quadriceps muscles. They extend, straighten your lower leg, and lift your thigh forward *(XI-B)*. In the back of your thighs are your three hamstrings *(XI-C)*. These muscles bend your lower legs up toward your thighs, lift your thigh back, and lift your pelvis back. You have long and short muscles on the outside and inside of your thighs that lift them out to each side and bring them back to or past your midline. These muscles cooperate to turn your entire leg in or out.

Since most of your thigh muscles pass two joints, and move your pelvis or your thigh or your lower leg, they sometimes have trouble if they are trying to do two jobs at once. For instance, your quadriceps has trouble lifting your thigh and extending your lower leg when it is also lifting your pelvis forward. If your pelvis is properly aligned up and down, then your quadriceps has more power to lift your thigh and extend your lower leg. Try this to experience the difference. Many of the exercises in this chapter direct you first to move your thighs in a bent position and then to extend your lower

XI-B

XI-C

legs. This lets you stretch and strengthen your muscles in the most efficient way, according to the way they are structured in your body.

The basic mechanical imbalances in your thighs often derive from the habit of locking your knees. (See Alignment in Chapter 15.) That creates tight hamstrings and relatively weak quadriceps. Locking your knees can also create serious problems for your lower back and contributes to detrimental habits of walking and running. The major muscle problems for your thighs often come from incorrect and inadequate stretching.

To handle this series of problems, the first step is to stretch and strengthen your thigh muscles correctly by using the exercises in this chapter, and then to learn the correct mechanics of standing and walking to solve and then prevent these problems from recurring. Guidelines to help you do this are in Chapter 3.

Those of you who are working on having "thin thighs" should turn to the thigh lifts in Chapter 12 (exercises 74, 75, 77 and 78). In addition, any activity in which your legs move sideways will work these unused muscles and contribute to their firmness. Of course, controlling calorie intake will also help: exercise can help firm your muscles but only burning stored fat will make them thinner.

Guidelines for relieving sore leg muscles and groin pain are found in Chapter 16.

Exercises

There are four areas of your thighs to be exercised; the front, the quadriceps muscles; the back, the hamstrings; the inner thigh; and the outer thigh. This chapter describes the stretching and strengthening exercises for your quadriceps and hamstrings; exercises for the inner and outer thigh are found in Chapter 12. The order of the exercises in this book is not always the order in which you should do them. For instance, you should do a quadriceps stretch before you do the Pretzel or the Open Tailor Sit (exercises 56, 54). And you might want to do a Pretzel before you do stretches for your hamstrings, though you will also find that after you do any of the hamstring stretches, it will be easier for you to get your upper body lower and get more stretch in the Pretzel. Chapter 3 describes how these exercises fit together.

61   SITTING QUADRICEPS STRETCH

This stretch is also known as a Modified Hurdler's Stretch. Use this stretch before doing the Pretzel or Open Tailor Sit (exercises 56, 54).

STARTING POSITION: Sit on the floor with your right leg bent and lying in front of you and that knee pointing to the right. The outside of that leg is lying on the floor. Bend your left leg and put it on your left side, with that knee pointing diagonally to your left. The inside of your left leg is down on the floor. Both of your knees are bent more than a right angle, *61a.* Do not bend your left leg so that you are almost sitting on it. The degree of bend should enable you to feel stretch in your quadriceps muscles and feel no discomfort in your knee. {**Troubleshooting:** Both of your knees should be comfortable and have no sensation in them at all. The position of your left foot is crucial to preventing knee injury while sitting in this stretch. Your foot should be extended and lying on its side (the inside). Do not forcefully point it and turn it over to be on its top. Do not flex it so that your foot is at a right angle to your lower leg. Both of these positions can cause you to misalign your leg bones at the knee joint. Make sure to adjust your foot so that you feel no discomfort in your knee, even if you actually need to flex your foot.}

The position of your upper body and your arms is also crucial to preventing lower back injury in this position. Rest down on your right forearm, diagonally back from the line of your left thigh. Put your left arm forward on your right knee or right lower leg. This arm position pulls your rib cage forward and prevents it from arching and straining your lower back. Keep your head aligned and your chin in. If this position hurts your back, then rest your upper body to your

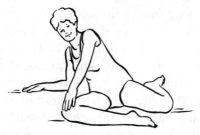

61a

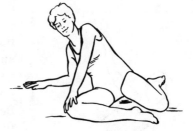

61b

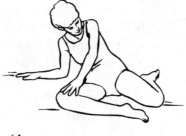

61c

right side and bring your left leg farther back (see exercise 64).

THE STRETCH: **(1)** By just putting your body into this position, you should be feeling a strong stretch in the muscles along the top of your left thigh. If you are not feeling the stretch, you need to gently press down your left buttock. You may not be able to lay it completely on the floor, but the action of pressing it down to the floor will produce the first part of this stretch. Hold this first position for 30 seconds to a minute. **(2)** Tighten the muscles under your left buttock and press up the front of your hip, *61b*. Turn your upper body so that you are looking down toward your supporting right arm and hold that position for 30 seconds to a minute. This is not much of a movement, but it will produce an increase in the stretch sensation that you feel in your thigh, especially across the top of your thigh. Hold this position for 30 seconds to a minute. Relax your buttock muscles and now **(3)** pull in your abdominal muscles, pull your rib cage up away from your waist, bring your chin in, and curve your head toward your left knee by tipping your forehead toward the thigh you are stretching, *61c*. This action pulls your up-

125

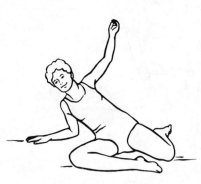

61d

per body away from your left thigh and makes the stretch sensation even stronger than it was before. Hold this position for 30 seconds to a minute. {**Troubleshooting:** If you feel any discomfort in your left knee during this stretch, you can sometimes eliminate the problem by lifting your left heel just a little. Or move your left leg out more to your left side.} Be sure to do the Salt Shaker (exercise 62) before you repeat this stretch on your right leg. Always finish the Sitting Quadriceps Stretch with the Salt Shaker. **(4)** Lift your left arm back, keeping your palm facing up, and let it sink down behind you. This arm position will stretch your shoulder in a somewhat milder way than the Shoulder Stretch from the Side (exercise 11) against the wall. The position of your arm is neither vertical, above your head, nor horizontal from your shoulder. It is in between these positions and is on a high diagonal, *61d*.

62   SALT SHAKER

After you have done the Sitting Quadriceps Stretch (exercise 61), in order to change sides and relax any tension in your lower back, do the Salt Shaker: Lift up your left leg by leading with your knee. Pretend your knee is the top of a salt shaker and pour out some salt on the outside of your right leg. When you are in Salt Shaker position, your left foot is pointing toward the ceiling and your lower leg is trying to be in a vertical line. Your left leg is reaching across your right thigh, *62*. Hold this position for 30 seconds to a minute. Now repeat the Sitting Quadriceps Stretch and then the Salt Shaker on your right leg.

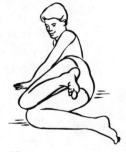

62

63

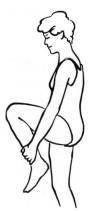

63a

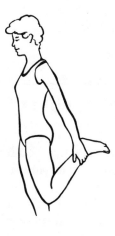

63b

STANDING QUADRICEPS STRETCH

This stretch is difficult to do for people who have a painful or potentially painful back condition. If you are one of these people, don't do this stretch.

STARTING POSITION: Stand where you can lean against a wall or hold on to something for balance. (You can also do the stretch without holding on to something.) Unlock your standing leg, your right. Your right foot should be pointing straight ahead. Hold in your abdominal muscles and align your head, with your chin in. Bend your left leg and lift your leg so that your knee is in front of you. Now reach with your left arm and take hold of your left ankle with your left hand, *63a.*

THE STRETCH: **(1)** Carefully bring your bent left leg behind you. Make sure that your knee is pointing straight down to the ground. Push your hand with your left foot and try to make a right angle at your knee with your lower leg and thigh, *63b.* This will produce a strong stretch in your quadriceps muscles. Hold this position for 30 seconds to a minute. {**Troubleshooting:** Be very careful here not to feel any pain or discomfort in your lower back. Bring your upper body forward from your waist to help prevent back strain. If your arms are too short to do this stretch without pain, don't do it. Another mistake you should not make is to squeeze your foot toward your buttocks, which stretches the ligaments in your knees.} **(2)** Now, just as in the Sitting Quadriceps Stretch (exercise 61), tighten your left buttock muscles and you will feel the stretch higher up in that group of muscles. This tightening also helps prevent back discomfort. Hold this position for 30 seconds to a minute. **(3)** Relax the tightening and curve your head down toward your left knee by bringing your chin in and tipping your forehead forward. This has the same result as in the Sitting Quadriceps Stretch. Hold this position for 30 seconds to a minute. Repeat this stretch on your right leg.

64

SIDE LYING QUADRICEPS STRETCH

If you have any lower back or knee pain when trying to do the previous quadriceps stretches, then you should try this one. It is the same as the Standing Quadriceps Stretch (exercise 63), except you are lying on your side.

STARTING POSITION: Lie on your right side. Rest your head on your bent arm, which cushions your head like a pillow. You can either extend your right leg or bend it. Hold in your abdominal muscles. Bend your left leg and bring your knee forward and up toward your chest, so that you can easily take hold of your left ankle with your left hand.

THE STRETCH: Your left hand brings your bent left leg back, so that you feel stretch in the front of your left thigh. The angle of your left thigh is just a little back from straight down from your hip socket. Keep pushing your foot into your hand and do *not* squeeze your heel toward your buttocks! Hold this position for 30 seconds to a minute. Now tighten your buttocks as though you were trying to tuck under your pelvis. Hold that position for 30 seconds to a minute. Repeat this stretch on your right leg.

65

QUADRICEPS STRETCH FOR PEOPLE WITH LOOSE LIGAMENTS

When you do any of these quadriceps stretches, you need to be extremely careful of your knees and your lower back. That care is especially important when doing this next stretch. People with loose ligaments have trouble feeling some stretches that most people feel easily. So this stretch is for you. Those of you who do not have the trouble of loose ligaments also can do this stretch. It is very strong and you must be very careful to follow the instructions to prevent knee injury.

STARTING POSITION: Kneel on all fours on the floor. Then bend your elbows and rest your weight down on your forearms. Slide your right knee back so that your right thigh is almost parallel to the floor, and keep your leg bent so that your right foot is pointing up to the ceiling or toward your

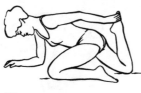

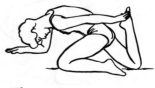

65a   65b

head. Reach back with your left arm and take hold of your right foot with your left hand. Hold your foot at any place that is comfortable, *65a*. {**Troubleshooting:** Sometimes it is hard to reach your foot and your hamstrings may start to cramp. Pull out the cramp before going on with this stretch. To insure that you are not going to hurt your left knee, make sure that your right forearm is directly under your right shoulder, so that you are supporting your weight on your right forearm and not resting too much of your weight on your left (potentially overbent) knee. Untuck the toes of your left foot. Keep your head aligned and your chin in.}

THE STRETCH: (1) Let your pelvis sink down toward the floor and slide your right leg back a little farther along the floor while holding on to your foot. Don't squeeze your knee; just hold your right foot in your left hand. This position has your weight on the muscles directly above your right knee and not on your knee bones themselves. Hold this position for 30 seconds to a minute. (3) Tighten your abdominal muscles and round your back up a little, *65b*. This new position makes the stretch even stronger. Hold this position for 30 seconds to a minute. Repeat this stretch on your left leg.

66   DEEP LUNGE

This is a strong stretch for the top front part of your thigh. It is also very helpful to do before you do the Standing Hamstring Stretch (exercise 71), because you are able to fold more easily at the hip socket. You must take care to protect your back while doing this.

STARTING POSITION: Stand and bend your knees so you can lean down and put both of your hands on the floor in front of your feet. Reach your right leg all the way back as far as it will extend. Keep your left leg bent at a right angle

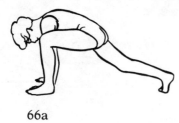

66a

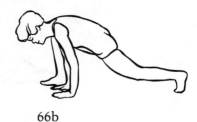

66b

only: that means that your lower leg is straight up from the floor and your thigh is at a right angle to it. If your knee is overbent and less than a right angle, you will be squeezing your knee too much and stretching your knee ligaments. To adjust this angle, reach your right leg farther back. Hold in your abdominal muscles, align your head, chin in, and keep both feet straight ahead.

THE STRETCH: **(1)** With your hands on the floor on both sides of your left bent leg, gently press your pelvis toward the floor, *66a*. This position gives you a strong stretch sensation across the top of your thigh at your hip socket. Hold this position for 30 seconds to a minute. **(2)** Now move your left hand to the inside of your left bent leg and allow your pelvis to sink lower. **(3)** Move your pelvis to the right and curve your head toward your left knee so your entire body is shaped like a banana, *66b*. You will feel the stretch farther toward the outside of the top of your right thigh. Hold this position for 30 seconds to a minute. {**Troubleshooting:** Do not feel any discomfort in either of your hip sockets during this stretch. If you do, move your upper body toward your extended leg and adjust the weight of your upper body back by moving your hands back. Make sure your feet are straight ahead and not turned in or out.}

Repeat this stretch on your left leg. To change legs, bend your right knee and put it down on the floor. Push your pelvis back so you are kneeling on all fours. Then put your right leg forward with your knee at a right angle. Now extend your left leg back and put your body into the lunge position.

This stretch also provides the second part of the preparation for the Splits (exercise 67). The Deep Lunge can be a very effective and challenging strengthening exercise. You will use it to strengthen your quadriceps muscles in Lifting Up from a Deep Lunge (exercise 70).

67

SPLITS

There are two parts to the preparation for doing the splits, which is, itself, a stretch. It stretches the hamstrings of your front leg and the top of the quadriceps of your back leg.

PRELIMINARY STARTING POSITION: Sit on the floor with your right leg extended in front of you, and your left leg bent and turned over so that the inside of your thigh is on the floor, *67a*. Place it as far back as you can. That may be only at a right angle to your extended right leg, or it may be a little diagonally back from the right angle. It is this bent left leg you will stretch first. Lean your upper body forward over your right leg, *67b*. Make sure that you are bending at the hip socket. If necessary, bend your right knee in order to bend forward correctly. Your right knee will not be straight up to the ceiling but will turn out a little to your right.

PRELIMINARY STRETCH: **(1)** You are going to move your bent left leg back farther than it is in the starting position. You will use your left foot in a manner very similar to the way a duck swims. Flex and then extend your foot two or three times. The action of your foot on the floor will pull your bent leg back. **(2)** Carefully lift your upper body up to almost a vertical position, *67c*. Hold this position for 30 seconds to a minute. You should feel a strong stretch on the top of your quadriceps muscles. {**Troubleshooting:** Be sure you do not feel any discomfort in your lower back. If you do, do not bring your upper body up quite so far.} **(3)** Bend your upper body down again and repeat the foot flex-and-extend movements of step 1. **(4)** Repeat step 2: That is, carefully bring up your upper body and hold that position for 30 seconds to a minute.

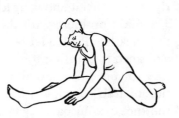

67a   67b   67c

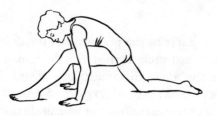

67d

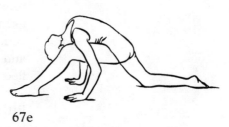

67e

Repeat this stretch sequence with your right leg bent behind you and your left extended in front of you.

Now do the Deep Lunge (exercise 66), first on one leg, then on the other. When you have completed these two preliminary stretches, you are ready to try the splits stretch itself.

STARTING POSITION: Get back into the Deep Lunge position, with your left leg bent in front and your right leg extended behind you. Place your left hand on the floor outside of your left leg and your right hand inside this leg. You will be holding your weight on your hands. Untuck the toes of your right foot so your weight is resting on the top of that foot. Take care to point your foot straight back, not in or out. *67d.*

THE STRETCH: Slowly extend your left leg forward and let your pelvis and your upper body sink down. Keep your upper body forward, *67e.* You will feel the strongest part of this stretch in your left hamstrings. Hold this position as long as you can tolerate the discomfort. When you have had enough of that stretch, bend your left (front) leg and gently sit down toward your left buttock.

Repeat this Splits stretch on the other side, with your right leg in front and your left leg in back. {**Troubleshooting:** The main problem with the splits occurs in the position of the back leg. People let it turn out so the inside of the thigh and knee is pointing toward the floor. This risks serious injury to your knee and allows your pelvis to get into a position to arch your lower back. By keeping the top or front of the knee of your back leg facing the floor, you will be stretching muscles and not hurting your back or knees.}

68

LEG EXTENSIONS

This exercise is a very effective way to strengthen your quadriceps so that you will have strength in the many positions in which you will need it.

STARTING POSITION: Stand near a wall or bar or something you can hold to maintain your balance. Hold on with your right hand extended out to your side. This series of exercises is similar to one dancers do at the bar. You can choose to hold on or not. Keep the foot of your supporting leg straight forward and your knee unlocked. Press down your toes to help stabilize your ankle. Hold in your abdominal muscles and align your head, with your chin in.

THE STRENGTHENING EXERCISE: **(1)** Bend your right leg and lift it up in front of you about 6 inches, *68a*, taking 4 counts. **(2)** Slowly extend your lower leg forward to a straight but not locked position, *68b,c*, taking 4 counts. **(3)** Bend your lower leg down to your starting position in 4 counts, but don't lower your thigh. **(4)** Lift your bent leg 3 to 4 inches in 4 counts. **(5)** Extend your lower leg forward to a straight but not locked position, taking 4 counts. **(6)** Bend your leg again without lowering your thigh, taking 4 counts. **(7)** Once more lift your bent leg 3 to 4 inches in 4 counts. **(8)** Extend your lower leg in 4 counts. **(9)** Lower your extended leg to the floor and put it down next to your left foot. Take 8 slow counts to do this.

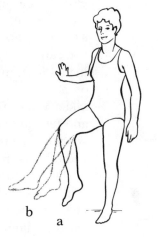

68   c   b   a

133

Repeat this sequence with your left leg lifting and extending and your right leg supporting you. You can repeat this sequence with your leg extending diagonally forward, out to your side, diagonally back, or directly back. {**Troubleshooting:** Take care not to lock the standing leg during this sequence, and keep your body weight distributed on the entire surface of your supporting foot, not only or mainly on your heel. The biggest difficulty occurs at the hip of the lifting and extending leg. You need to keep your hip level. Your hip naturally lifts when you lift your leg. You must consciously put it back where it is even with the hip of your standing leg, or you might feel discomfort in the hip joint. Keeping your hips level is even more difficult as you extend your leg in different directions around your body. When you extend your leg diagonally back and straight back, tip your entire upper body forward about 4 to 6 inches in order to prevent back injury. Only lift your leg as high toward the rear as it will go without arching your lower back. When you are extending your leg back, you are strengthening your hamstrings.}

69

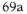
69a

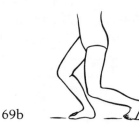
69b

ALMOST KNEELING

This is another exercise to strengthen your quadriceps muscles. It is a little more strenuous than Leg Extensions (exercise 68), because you are lowering and lifting more weight with the muscles you are strengthening.

STARTING POSITION: Stand near a wall or something that you can hold on to for balance. Place one foot about 12 to 14 inches in front of the other. Do *not* pretend you are standing on a line, but place your foot forward as though you had taken a step. Transfer your weight forward to your front foot and let the heel of your back foot come off the floor. Align your upper body so that your ears are over your shoulders, your chin is in, your jaw is relaxed, your shoulder blades are down and back, and your abdominal muscles are held in, *69a.*

THE STRENGTHENING EXERCISE: (1) Slowly bend your knees as though the knee of the back leg were going to touch the floor, *69b,c.* Keep your weight over your front leg, and

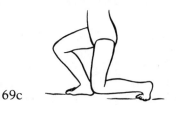

69c

feel most of the work happening in that thigh. Do not let that back knee touch the floor, and do not let the heel of your front foot come off the floor. Take 8 counts to do this. Keep your upper body as upright as is comfortable, though it may come forward a little. **(2)** Slowly lift your body up again by straightening your legs in 8 counts. Repeat the lowering and lifting three more times and then repeat the exercise on the other side with your back leg now in front.

70 LIFTING UP FROM A DEEP LUNGE

This exercise is very strenuous. It is very good for building the kind of quadriceps strength that football players and competitive weightlifters need. If you do not need that kind of strength, you do not need to do it.

STARTING POSITION: Put your body into the stretch position of Deep Lunge (exercise 66). Extend your arms out to your sides. Align your head, with your chin in, and hold in your abdominal muscles, *70a*.

THE STRENGTHENING EXERCISE: Slowly extend your bent front leg and bring yourself up to a standing position, *70b,c*. To start this movement, you will need to transfer your weight from being distributed on both of your feet to its being primarily on your bent front leg. Lean your upper body forward a little to start to pull your back leg forward as you straighten your front leg. Take 8 slow counts to do this. Repeat this exercise with your legs in opposite positions. {**Troubleshooting:** To protect your back, keep your upper body forward. To protect your front knee, make sure that you keep your heel on the floor to prevent it from overbending.}

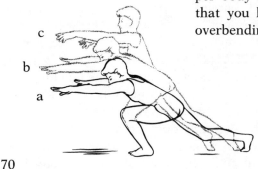

c

b

a

70

71

STANDING HAMSTRING STRETCH

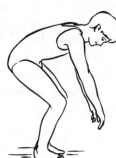

71a

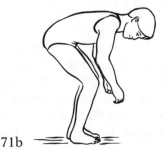

71b

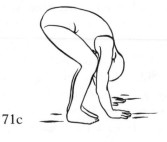

71c

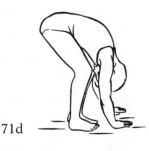

71d

Your hamstring muscles are often very tight because of how much work they do to help keep your body upright all day long. There are three positions for stretching these muscles: standing, lying down, and sitting. If you have very tight hamstrings or have a back injury, you should do the lying down stretch first and then the standing and sitting parts. After completing all of the parts of this stretch exercise, your legs should move much more freely when you walk, run, or do any of the other activities you do each day. Before you stretch your hamstrings, *always* stretch your calf muscles so that you will be able to concentrate on the sensation of your hamstrings stretching. If your calf muscles are tight or un-stretched you will primarily feel them stretching and not your hamstrings. If at any time you feel pain in your hip socket during these hamstring stretches, do not do them. See Troubleshooting at the end of page 72.

STARTING POSITION: Before you bend your upper body down and put your hands on the floor, you need to: **(1)** Place your feet straight forward and 4 to 6 inches apart to be directly under their hip sockets. **(2)** Hold in your abdominal muscles and stretch up your waist. **(3)** Bend your knees a lot. **(4)** Align your head and relax your jaw. Now you are ready to **(5)** fold your upper body forward at your hip sockets, *71a,b.* Bending over in this position protects your lower back. When your upper body is hanging down, put your hands on the floor in front of your feet and let your head hang down, *71c.* If the backs of your thighs are so tight in this position that you are almost squatting, place a telephone book or two under your palms.

THE STRETCH: **(1)** Carefully start to straighten one leg and hold it partially straight for 6 to 10 counts. Keep your rib cage touching the thigh of the leg that you are partially straightening, *71d.* **(2)** Relax that leg and partially straighten your other leg. Keep your rib cage touching your thigh. Hold this position for 6 to 10 counts. {**Troubleshooting:** Aim to have your buttocks pointing up toward the ceiling. Keep your elbows from straightening. If you straighten your elbows, you will separate your rib cage from your thighs and prevent the weight of your upper body from hanging down and stretching your hamstrings. Your legs do not need to be entirely straightened to stretch your hamstrings. If you feel pain directly behind your knee, or feel no stretch sensation in your hamstrings but feel a very strong stretch in your calves, then put a ¾- to 2-inch-high book under just your heels. This will compensate for your very tight calf muscles and let you stretch your hamstrings. You need to do the Phone Book Calf Stretch (exercise 88).}

(3) Now move both your hands in front of the first leg you stretched and repeat the unbending process. {**Troubleshooting:** Keep your elbows relaxed and lean on the floor on your hands. Don't push away from the floor. Let your head relax and hang down; don't pull it toward your leg.} Hold this position for 6 to 10 counts. Now relax the first leg and (4) move your hands in front of the other leg and repeat the unbending process with relaxed elbows. After 6 to 10 counts, relax the second leg and (5) move your hands to the outside of your first leg and put your little finger next to your little toe and unbend that leg, *71e.* Let your head hang down from your neck. Hold that position for 6 to 10 counts. (6) Relax that leg and move your hands to the outside of your other leg, little finger next to little toe. Unbend that leg and hold for 6 to 10 counts. During this entire sequence, keep your upper body touching the thigh of the leg you are unbending.

If you need to stand up because you've been upside-down too long, do so this way: keep your legs bent; hold in your abdominal muscles and bring your upper body to a vertical position; then straighten your legs. This way of standing up and bending down protects the lumbar area of your spine from strain and prevents very painful back trouble, which can be triggered when you bend forward over straightened or locked legs with your abdominal muscles passive. Rest a few seconds and then bend down again the same way you did before.

After you have stretched both of your legs, one at a time, three times, you are now ready to stretch both at the same time. (7) With your legs still bent, rock forward so that you feel some of your weight on your palms, *71f.* You need to keep your chest touching your thighs. Now unbend both of your legs as far as you can with your upper body touching your thighs. Be sure not to straighten your elbows because

71e

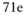
71f

137

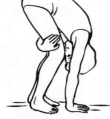

71g

then you lift your upper body and the traction effect no longer can help stretch your muscles. The stretch sensation in your hamstrings should be very strong. Hold this position for 6 to 10 counts. **(8)** Transfer your weight back to your feet, and hug your left arm around your legs and move your right hand in front of both your feet. Don't let your knees come together. By hugging your thighs and bringing your upper body closer to your thighs, you transfer more of your weight forward and down. This stretches your hamstrings more effectively. **(9)** Rock forward so that you are holding some of your weight on your right hand, and unbend both of your legs again, keeping your upper body touching your thighs, *71g*. Hold this position for 6 to 10 counts. {**Troubleshooting:** Don't let your knees close together; keep them apart and over your feet.} **(10)** Rock back so your weight is mainly on your feet and switch the arms that are doing the hugging and supporting. **(11)** Rock your weight forward so that your right hand is supporting your weight, and unbend both of your legs, keeping your upper body touching your thigh. Hold this position for 6 to 10 counts. **(12)** Rock your weight back onto your feet, bend your knees a lot, and sit down.

72

TRIPLE HAMSTRING STRETCH

Your hamstrings are a strong and very tight group of muscles. This next sequence can help increase their flexibility even after completing the Standing Hamstring Stretch (exercise 71).

LYING DOWN

STARTING POSITION: Lie on your back. Bend your right leg and bring your thigh as close to your pelvis as possible. Now move your bent leg to the right so it is next to your pelvis and not on top of it. You knee is near your right shoulder. Extend your left leg straight down.

THE STRETCH: **(1)** Hug your thigh with your right arm or both arms and then unbend your lower leg as far as you can, *72a*. Use your arm strength to keep your leg as close to your body as possible. Hold this position for 30 seconds to a minute. **(2)** Move your hands up to your calf and continue to pull your extended leg toward your right armpit, *72e*. Hold this position for 30 seconds to a minute. {**Troubleshooting:** It is

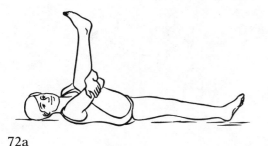

72a

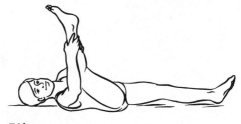

72b

SITTING

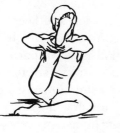

72c

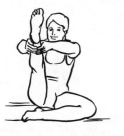

72d

important to keep your thigh touching the side of your pelvis. It is *not* important to straighten out your leg to a straight line. What is of utmost importance is that you feel a stretch sensation in your hamstrings.}

You will need to sit up to do the next part of the stretch. To do this, stop hugging your right leg and bend it. Bend your left leg and put it next to your bent right leg. Roll to your right side and use your arms to push yourself up to a sitting position. If you sit up this way, by rolling to one side or the other, you prevent strain on your lower back.

STARTING POSITION: You are going to continue to stretch your right leg. Sit with your left leg bent in front of you, with the outside of your thigh resting on the floor. This bent-leg position helps you balance while sitting in this stretch position. Bend and lift your right leg. Hold it with both of your hands around your calf. Keep your thigh close to your pelvis and lift your right buttock off the floor. You are now sitting on your left buttock and the side of your bent left leg.

THE STRETCH: **(1)** With your right buttock lifted off the floor, gently lift your extended right leg higher up toward your shoulder, *72c*. Hold this position for 30 seconds to a minute. **(2)** Carefully sit your right buttock down on the floor while still holding your leg up. Hold in your abdominal muscles, *72d*. When you sit down on this buttock, the stretch feeling is much stronger. Hold this position for 30 seconds to a minute. {**Troubleshooting:** Do not try to straighten your leg entirely. Allow your knee to be softly bent during this stretching so that you feel stretch only in your hamstring muscles and feel *no* strain in your lower back or behind your knee. Make sure that your leg is not rotated in or out, even when your hip is off the floor.}

139

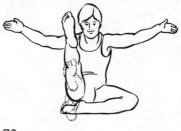

72e

(3) Now let go of your leg and try to keep your leg as high as it was when your hands were holding it. Slowly lower your leg to the floor, *72e*. Keep it extended, straightened but not locked (not hyperextended). Take 8 slow counts to lower your leg to the floor.

SITTING BENT FORWARD

Here is the last part of this sequence. You are going to do one more final stretch for your right leg.

STARTING POSITION: Bend both of your legs. You will be stretching only your right one. Bend your upper body forward at your hip sockets. Sit so far forward that you feel your weight in front of your sitz bones. Your thighs and pelvis will again be touching. Wrap one or both of your arms under and around your right leg and hug your leg so that your pelvis and upper body stay attached, *72f*.

THE STRETCH: Unbend your right leg and keep your upper body touching your leg, *72g*. You may not be able to straighten your leg entirely and that is not important. What is important is that you feel this strong stretch in your hamstring muscles. Reach your head down your leg as though the top of your head could touch your toes. Hold this position until the tightness in your hamstring relaxes, from 30 seconds to a minute. While you keep your right arm un-

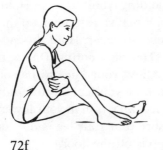

72f

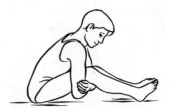

72g

der your right leg, reach your left hand down and press on the top of your right foot to extend your ankle and point your toes. This gives the top of your foot a strong stretch. Keep your other (left) leg bent and that knee up.

Note: Whenever you do any exercises sitting on the floor with your legs extended in front or to the sides, keep your heels on the floor. When you lift up your heels, you lock (hyperextend) your knees, and that harms your knees.

Now you are ready to repeat this sequence on your left leg. You will do the Hamstring Stretch lying down, *72a,b*, then you will sit up and do it sitting, *72c,d,e*, and finally you will do it sitting bent forward, *72f,g*. When you have completed this sequence on your left leg, stand up and do the final steps of the Standing Hamstring Stretch (exercise 71), with both legs unbending. Your muscles should now be very much more stretched than before you did the lying down and sitting stretches, and you might be able to reach your hands back behind your feet.

{**Troubleshooting:** When repeating the standing stretch, you need to keep your weight down on your hands, so keep your elbows bent and relaxed. If you hug both of your arms around your legs, you will be causing two counterproductive things to happen: your upper body will stop touching your lower body and that might hurt your lower back; the weight of your upper body will stop hanging down, which will eliminate the traction effect and reduce the stretching. If you have pain in your hip sockets during these stretches, you need to stretch your hamstrings by standing and placing one leg on a table the height of your leg. Place your standing leg back, beyond a vertical line and be sure not to lock your knee. Then follow all the directions in part three of 72. You may want to place your upper body inside your stretching leg and not directly over it to prevent any pain in your hip socket. After about six weeks of daily stretching in this position, you may be able to stretch your hamstrings in the other positions in 71 and 72.}

73   BACKWARD LEG CIRCLES

You are strengthening your hamstrings when you are doing Leg Extensions with your leg extended diagonally back or

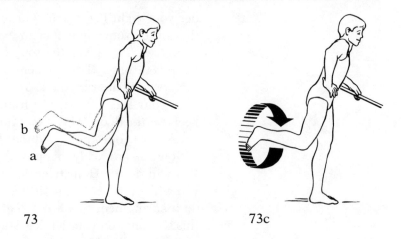

73   73c

directly back. Here is another simple way to strengthen your hamstrings.

STARTING POSITION: Stand where you can lean on a bar, wall or counter. Your support can be in front of you or to either side. Align your head over your shoulders, with your chin in. Hold in your abdominal muscles. You will be working with one leg at a time and you need to keep the knee of your supporting leg unlocked.

THE STRENGTHENING EXERCISE: **(1)** Bend your right leg and lift it up about 6 to 8 inches behind you, *73a,b*. Take 4 counts to do this. **(2)** Slowly lift up your leg 4 inches, taking 4 counts. **(3)** Lower it 4 inches, *73a*, in 4 counts. Repeat steps 2 and 3, three more times. **(4)** Slowly draw a 6-inch-circumference circle behind you, *73c*, taking 8 to 10 counts. **(5)** Now draw another circle with your knee and have your circle go in the opposite direction. Take 8 to 10 counts to do this. **(6)** Lower your leg to the floor in 4 counts. Repeat this sequence with your left leg.

When you have completed this exercise, take a few minutes to do the Standing Hamstring Stretch (exercise 71). Then you can repeat this sequence with your lifted leg in an extended position instead of a bent position. {**Troubleshooting:** To protect your lower back, let your upper body tip forward 4 to 6 inches. Don't lift your leg so high that you feel discomfort in your lower back. You can increase the height your leg can lift by doing any quadriceps stretch (exercises 61–65) and the Deep Lunge (exercise 66).}

12 Your Thighs: Inner and Outer

So far, the order of the exercises in this book has been first the stretching and then the strengthening ones. This chapter will reverse the usual order because the strengthening exercises will enable you to stretch some of these muscle groups more easily. That is why the inner thigh exercises are in the order that follows. Your thigh muscles are shown in illustrations *XII-A* (outer thigh) and *XII-B* (inner thigh).

Some of the stretches in this chapter have several parts. You can choose to do just the first part or proceed to the others. Dancers, gymnasts, and anyone else who needs extreme flexibility should follow the entire series.

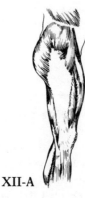

XII-A

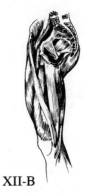

XII-B

Exercises

74   INNER THIGH LIFTS

STARTING POSITION: Lie on your right side. Rest your head on your bent right arm so it is comfortable. Bend your left leg and put your left foot on the floor in front of your right thigh, above the knee. Your left knee is pointing up to the ceiling. Rest your left hand on the floor in front of your chest and use it to help you remain balanced on your side, or hold on to your left ankle, *74a*.

THE STRENGTHENING EXERCISE: **(1)** Lift up your right leg and keep your knee facing forward. You will feel your inner thigh muscles working as they lift your leg. Take 4 slow counts to do this. **(2)** Lower your leg to the floor, *74b,c*. Keep your leg extended but make sure not to lock your knee. Repeat this lift-and-lower pattern three more times. You may not be able to lift your leg very high when you first start this exercise. Over time, you will be able to lift it higher, though you will find there is a limited range because of the position of your legs. Repeat this exercise on your left side for your left inner thigh.

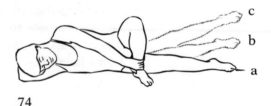

74

75   INNER AND OUTER THIGH LIFTS

This exercise is more strenuous than Inner Thigh Lifts (exercise 74) and gets your inner thighs ready for stretching a little more effectively. When you no longer feel challenged by Inner Thigh Lifts, you are ready for this exercise.

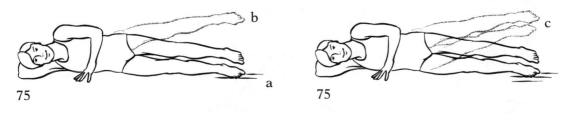

75

75

STARTING POSITION: Lie on your right side as you did for Inner Thigh Lifts, but extend both of your legs. Place your left hand about 10 inches in front of your chest to help you balance and keep your body on its side. *75a.*

THE STRENGTHENING EXERCISE: **(1)** Lift up your left leg as high as it can go and still keep your knee forward, *75b.* Do not turn it so that your knee is facing the ceiling. Take 4 counts to lift your leg. **(2)** Lift your right leg just as you did in the Inner Thigh Lifts, taking 4 counts, *75c.* You will probably be able to lift it a little higher than you did for that exercise. **(3)** Lower your right leg to the floor in 4 counts. **(4)** Lower your left leg in 4 counts. Repeat this sequence three more times and then roll over and repeat it on your left side. {**Troubleshooting:** Hold in your abdominal muscles and make sure to lean on your supporting hand in order to keep your body on its side. It is a challenge to keep from rolling back a little.}

76   THREE-PART INNER THIGH STRETCH

CENTER

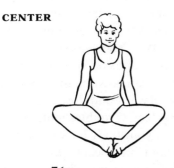

76a

Before you do any inner or outer thigh stretches, make sure you have stretched your calves, hamstrings, and quadriceps and done the Pretzel (exercise 56) for your buttock muscles. This stretch includes three parts: center, reaching, and final.

STARTING POSITION: Sit on the floor. Bend your knees so you can put the bottoms of your feet together, and let your legs fall open to each side. Do not pull your feet in toward your body; just put them on the floor where they go naturally. The shape of your legs in this position is a diamond. Put your hands on the floor 5 to 10 inches behind your hips. *76a.*

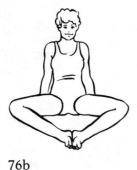

76b

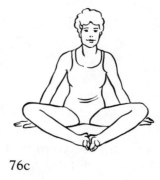

76c

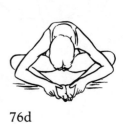

76d

THE STRETCH: There are several parts to the stretch so the sequence of the positions will be numbered. **(1)** Rock your legs to the right so that your right leg is on the floor. Now lift your hips off the floor and shift your body weight back on your hands. Your upper body is now on a backward diagonal. Allow the weight of your left leg to fall open to the left and let your feet open like a book with its pages open on the floor. Hold that position for 30 seconds, *76b*. Sit your hips down and rock your legs to the left so that your left leg is on the floor. Now lift your hips off the floor and allow the weight of your right leg to open to the right and hold this position for 30 seconds. When you stretch one side this way and then the other, you will feel the stretch on the upper leg much more strongly than the other. Now let your right leg pull your legs into an even position so both knees are an equal distance from the floor. Let the bottoms of your feet fall open and feel that your knees have small weights on them pulling them down. Hold this position for 30 seconds more. **(2)** Rest your hips back down on the floor. Lift your knees about 2 to 4 inches, and slide your feet about 2 to 3 inches forward along the floor. Then bend your upper body forward at your hip sockets. *76c*. With your elbows in front of your legs, not on them, put your hands on your ankles or hold on to your arches (don't hold on to your toes or pull them up). Pull your upper body forward and down as if the top of your head could touch your feet. {**Troubleshooting:** To protect your back, be sure to bend your body forward at the place where your leg goes into your hip socket. Don't bend forward from your waistline. Also, make sure to hold in your

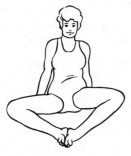

76e

abdominal muscles.} Your elbows should be pointing side-ways, not back toward your thighs. Make sure to move your elbows in front of your legs as you actively pull your upper body down, *76d.* Hold that position for 30 seconds to a min-ute. If you can't get your head close to your feet, then lift up your upper body a little and slide your feet forward 1 to 2 inches more. This will allow you to get your head lower. **(3)** Sit up. Lift your hips off the floor and shift your body weight back on your hands. Your upper body is now on a backward diagonal. Allow the bottoms of your feet to fall open like a book open on the floor and feel as if you had small weights on your knees, *76e.* You should feel a strong stretch along your inner thigh muscles. Hold this position for 30 seconds to a minute. **(4)** Sit your hips down on the floor again, and repeat step 2, pulling your upper body down to try to touch your head to your feet, *76c and d.* Hold this lowered position for 30 seconds to a minute.

If you are loose ligamented, you may not feel the stretch of this initial hip lift. You need to experiment with your leg position. Try separating your feet 4 to 6 inches before you lift your pelvis. Or move your feet forward still closed to-gether, so your legs are in a diamond before you lift your pelvis. You can place a 2- to 3-inch book under each of your lower legs or even cross your feet a little with them sup-ported in this way. When you pull your upper body forward (steps 2 and 4), it helps to put a folded towel or soft pad 1 to 2 inches thick under your thighs close to your buttocks. These supports enable you actually to feel the stretch in your muscles and not feel any discomfort in the ligaments at the front or back of your hip socket. Be sure to hold in your abdominal muscles to prevent any back discomfort.

The next two parts of the inner thigh stretch are for you who need a wide range of flexibility. For the next part of this stretch, you need another starting position.

STARTING POSITION: Move your left leg out to the side by straightening it and lifting it to your left side, or by sliding it to your left and then extending it on the floor. Turn your upper body so that you are now looking over your right leg. Your upper body has made a quarter turn to the right, *76f.* Bend your upper body down and rest it over your bent leg, supporting your weight on your right forearm. Do not rest

REACHING

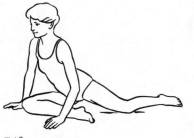

76f

your upper body down on your thigh and do not transfer your weight off your buttock. During the entire next part, do not allow your weight to transfer in front of your upper thigh bone that you feel resting on the floor. Now you need to adjust both of your legs. Move your right leg so that your knee is under your right armpit. Let your left leg reach behind you a little more than it was when you turned your upper body at first. Let your left knee be entirely relaxed on the floor. The inside of your left leg is on the floor and your leg is bent, not straightened. Now make sure that your right elbow is near the middle of your right thigh. Do not let your

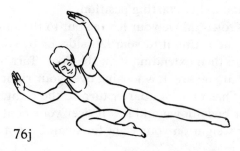

76g

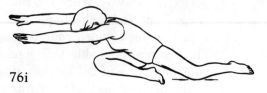

76h

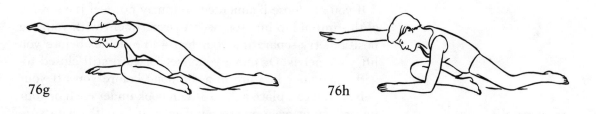

76i

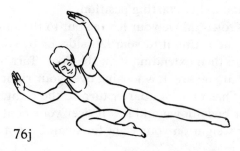

76j

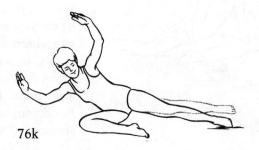

76k

upper body rest down on your thigh. Extend your head out from your neck and keep your chin in.

THE EXERCISE: **(1)** Reach out your left arm parallel to the floor over your bent right leg. Keep your head aligned and your chin in, *76g*. Hold this position for 30 seconds. Relax your legs and feel stretch just in your rib cage. **(2)** Now put your left arm down on the floor in front of your bent right leg, elbow near the middle of your shin, and reach out your right arm parallel to the floor in the same way that you did in step 1. Continue to keep your legs relaxed and feel stretch in your rib cage, *76h*. Hold this position for 30 seconds. **(3)** You are now going to do some abdominal muscle strengthening. To prepare, hold in your abdominal muscles and keep your chin in. Also, don't grit your teeth. Now lift up your left arm and hold it in the reaching position your right arm is in, *76i*. Hold this position for 4 counts. **(4)** Now rotate your entire upper body so that your left armpit is up to the ceiling, rather than your back as in step 7. You are facing the same direction as your right foot. Hold this position for 4 counts. **(5)** Now rotate your upper body down, *76j*, so you are in the same position as you were before you turned forward as in step 3. **(6)** Now again rotate your body to face forward as in step 4, and lift your extended left leg up about 3 to 4 inches above the floor, *76k*. This is very hard to do. Hold in your abdominal muscles and do not grit your teeth. Hold that position for 4 to 8 counts. (The stronger you get, the easier it will be to hold the position.) **(7)** Bring your left leg forward into the first inner thigh stretch position, with the bottoms of your feet together and your bent legs in the shape of a diamond. **(8)** Pull your upper body down to try to touch your head to your feet. Your upper body should be much lower than it was in *76d*. You should also feel that your left leg is lower to the floor than it was before you did this last sequence.

Repeat steps 1 through 8 on the other side, with your left leg bent and your right leg extended out to your left.

FINAL

STARTING POSITION: Assume the same position that you did for the center part of the exercise, with the bottoms of your feet together and your legs in a diamond shape.

THE STRETCH: **(1)** Pull your upper body down over your bent legs. If your head is very near your feet, turn your head

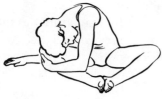

76l

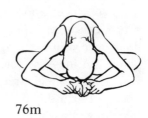

76m

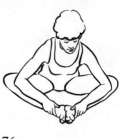

76n

sideways so the side of your forehead is near your feet. This position will let you pull your head a little lower. **(2)** Move your head toward your right knee, following the path of your bent right leg with your nose. Use your right hand on the floor behind your hips to help you move your body toward your knee, *76l*. Hold this position for 20 to 30 seconds. **(3)** Let your head come back over your feet. You should be able to pull your head even closer to your feet, *76m*. **(4)** Repeat step 2 to your left. Hold your head near your left knee for 20 to 30 seconds. **(5)** Return your body to the starting position, and pull your head down to your feet, *76m*. **(6)** Now place your forearms on your lower legs and gently press your legs down with your arms, *76n*. Hold this position for 30 seconds to a minute. **(7)** Release the pressure of your forearms and hold your legs open only with the muscles on the outside of your thighs (the part of your thighs most on thj floor right now), and bring your upper body up to a vertical position. Take 4 counts to do this. Relax your outer thigh muscles for a few seconds, and then without using your forearms to press down your legs, again contract these muscles (the "turnout" muscles for dancers) and bring your thighs closer to the floor. Hold this position for 4 counts or longer.

If you are unable to sit tailor fashion (with your legs crossed) because your inner thigh muscles are too tight, this stretch will enable you to gain comfort in that position. This stretch also gets your legs ready to stretch in the straddle sitting position in exercise 79. That stretch is good for anyone who needs a wide range of flexibility.

77

OUTER THIGH LIFTS, LYING

STARTING POSITION: Lie on the floor on your right side. Rest your head on your bent right arm. Bend your right leg to enable you to stay completely on your side. During this exercise you will need to hold in your abdominal muscles, keep your head aligned, with your chin in, and remember not to grit your teeth. You can use your left hand on the floor about 10 inches in front of your chest to help balance your body on its side, *77a*.

THE STRENGTHENING EXERCISE: **(1)** Slowly lift your left leg, taking 4 counts. Keep your knee unlocked and facing forward so that the side of your thigh does the lifting, *77b,c*. {**Troubleshooting:** Don't turn your leg so that your knee is up toward the ceiling, because then your quadriceps muscles are doing the lifting. Make sure to keep your foot gently extended; don't point it down to the floor, because that will cause joint pain in your hip socket.} **(2)** Slowly lower your leg to the floor in 4 counts. Repeat this lifting and lowering sequence seven more times. You can vary this sequence in this way: After you have lifted your leg **(3)** bend your leg in 4 slow counts and then **(4)** extend it in 4 slow counts. Then you can lower it as in step 2 above. You may not be able to repeat the sequence eight times, so just try for four or six repetitions. You can also vary the place where you start to lift your leg. Instead of starting with your leg extended in line with your body, put your leg forward, in front of your body, so that your leg and body are at a right angle. Repeat the same sequence: steps 1–2 — lift and lower — or 1,3,4,2 — lift, bend, straighten, and lower. Roll to your left side and repeat this exercise on your right leg. When you finish this, make sure to do the Pretzel stretch (exercise 56) until the tightness in your outer thigh muscles is pulled out.

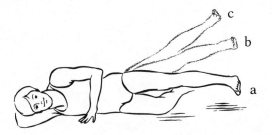

77

78

OUTER THIGH LIFTS, SITTING

STARTING POSITION: Sit on the floor with your legs bent and your feet to your left. Your knees are directly in front of your body. Lean your upper body forward and put your hands down on the floor. This position will transfer your weight onto your entire right thigh. This is important, because you do not want to have your weight back on only your buttocks. Your right hand will be a few inches in front of your knees and your left will be about 6 inches to the left of your right hand. Hold in your abdominal muscles and keep your head aligned and your chin in. *78a.*

THE STRENGTHENING EXERCISE: **(1)** Lift your bent left leg up about 3 inches and hold it there for 4 slow counts, *78b.* **(2)** Now lift your left leg up 2 to 3 more inches, *78c.* Do this in 2 slow counts and **(3)** lower your leg only 2 to 3 inches in 2 slow counts, *78b.* Repeat this lifting up in 2 counts, lowering a little in 2 counts, three more times. **(4)** Extend your jleg diagonally to the side in front. Do not have it straight to your side. Keep your knee forward and don't turn it up to the ceiling, *78d.* Repeat the 2- to 3-inch lift for 2 counts and the 2- to 3-inch lowering for 2 counts, four times, *78e,d.* **(5)** Bring your tired left leg around in front of your body without its touching the floor, and bend your upper body forward a little, *78f.* This is to stretch out your upper back. Rest your leg down on the floor and change sides. Repeat this sequence for your right leg, with your feet to your right side and your left thigh on the floor. {**Troubleshooting:** When you lift your bent leg, make sure to keep it in front of you. Also make sure

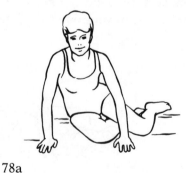

78a

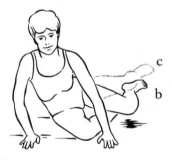

78

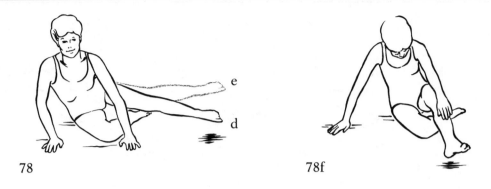

78   78f

to lift your entire leg, not just your knee. If you think of lifting your heel, you will be able to lift your entire leg. Do not feel any pain directly in your hip socket. If you do feel that pain, your knee is pointing either down or up too far, so adjust your thigh so that it is flat. You may need to bring your working leg forward more when you are lifting it to prevent any joint discomfort.} This strengthening is very good to do before you do the sitting part of the Straddle Stretch (exercise 79), because some of the muscles that you need to stretch here get very tired and then they relax more completely.

79

THREE-PART STRADDLE STRETCH

A three-part sequence of positions is necessary to stretch your inner thigh muscles in a straddle. The structure of this sequence is similar to the one you just did for the Inner Thigh Stretch (exercise 76). By doing this stretch after doing the Inner Thigh Stretch, your muscles will gain a great deal of flexibility. There are three parts to the exercise: sitting, upside-down, and final straddle.

SITTING

STARTING POSITION: Sit on the floor with your legs extended diagonally sideways. Place your legs only where they go naturally and do not force them to go wider apart than is comfortable. Bend your right leg, knee up toward the ceiling, and move your foot along the line created by your leg so that you can put your entire foot down on the floor. You

153

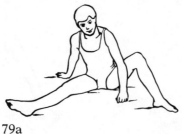

79a

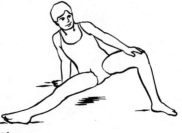

79b

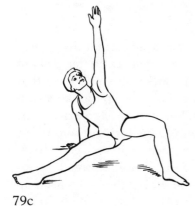

79c

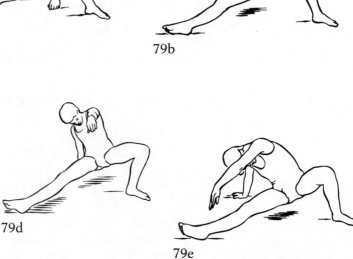

79d

79e

have moved your foot in and placed it on the floor about where the back of your knee was when it rested on the floor. Put your left hand on the floor 8 to 10 inches behind the middle of your left thigh. *79a.*

THE STRETCH: **(1)** Lift your pelvis up off the floor about 4 to 6 inches and have your weight on the outside of your left calf. This means you need to tuck your buttocks under a little to allow your entire left leg to turn out. Your left foot will rotate back and you will not have any weight on your heel. You should feel a mild stretch in your inner thigh muscles of your left leg, *79b.* To feel this stretch more, you can do the following: **(2)** Reach your right arm up to the ceiling in a long vertical line. At the same time, let the weight of your pelvis gently pull down, *79c.* **(3)** Curve your upper body forward at your rib cage, and reach your arm out in front of you, *79d.* **(4)** Now reach your right arm toward your left foot and allow your left leg to slide out along the floor 2 inches farther than it was, *79e.* In each of these positions, hold 20 to 30 seconds to feel the mild stretch. Sit back down on the floor and repeat this pelvis-lifted position on your other side. Your left leg is bent; your left foot is on the floor, and your right leg is rotated out and extended.

UPSIDE-DOWN

STARTING POSITION: Lie on your back. Bend your legs and bring your knees up and out on opposite diagonals toward your shoulders. You will stretch your right leg first, so put your left hand on your left knee and hold your left hip on the floor. Extend your right leg up and out so that it is reaching toward your right shoulder, *79f.* Before you do steps 1 and 2 of the stretch, use your extended leg to slowly draw two circles 8 inches in circumference, the first counterclockwise and the second clockwise, *79g.* Keep your leg extended toward your armpit. This is a mild strengthening exercise and it helps tire your inner thigh muscles so they will stretch more easily.

THE STRETCH: **(1)** Put your right hand on your right calf and pull your entire leg toward the floor, *79h.* This pull will lift your buttocks off the floor a little and that should happen. Hold this stretch for 30 seconds to a minute. Your right leg is *not* at a right angle to your pelvis but is reaching on a diagonal. You are reproducing the angle that your legs made when you were sitting on the floor but you are lying on your back. This diagonal position is important because you will feel the stretch along your inner thigh muscles. {**Troubleshooting:** If your leg is at a right angle to your pelvis, you will feel discomfort at the joint in your groin, and that is the kind of sensation you should not feel when doing these stretches.} **(2)** Repeat this stretch on your left leg. Bend your right leg and hold your right hand on your right knee. Extend your left leg toward your left shoulder and use your left

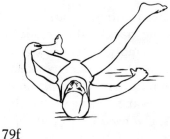

79f

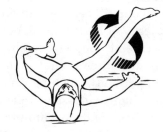

79g

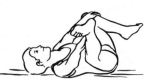

79h
(front view)

79h
(side view)

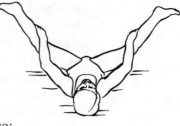

79i

hand to gently pull your left leg toward the floor after you do your leg circles. Hold this stretch position for 30 seconds to a minute. **(3)** Now extend your right leg again and gently pull down on both of your legs, *79i*. Hold this position for 30 seconds to a minute. **(4)** You are now going to close your legs together and at the same time use your hands to prevent your legs from closing. Begin to close your legs together and use your hands to push out on your legs where you are holding them at your calves. Your closing legs should be above your face and your legs are on a diagonal. They are not vertical. Take 6 to 8 counts to do this. Then sit up by first bending both of your legs and allowing them to roll you sideways. Sitting up from either side is a way to protect your back from strain.

FINAL STRADDLE

STARTING POSITION: The starting position is similar to the one you assumed for the sitting part of the Straddle Stretch. Sit with your legs comfortably extended wide apart. Turn and face your right leg, and bend your right knee so that you can wrap your arms around your right thigh and have your entire upper body — pelvis and rib cage — touching your thigh. In order to do this, you need to tip your upper body over toward your right leg. Your upper body is not bent at the waist, but your spine is extended and you feel that you are stretched up at the waist.

THE STRETCH: **(1)** While hugging your rib cage and thigh together, slowly extend your right leg, *79j*. Keep your upper body glued to your thigh as you extend your leg. In this stretch it is not necessary ever to straighten your leg entirely. It is necessary to keep your upper body touching your thigh. You will feel stretch in your hamstrings and inner thigh muscles. Hold this position for 30 seconds to a minute. When doing this stretch this way, your weight will not be on

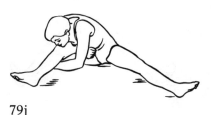

79j

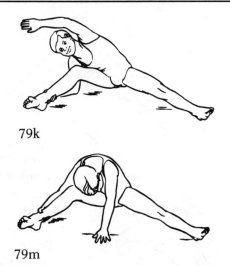

79k

79l

79m

both of your sitz bones. Your weight will be in front of your right sitz bone, and *your left buttock will come off the floor. Let this happen* because it prevents back injury and allows you to safely and effectively stretch these muscles. **(2)** Now turn your upper body a quarter turn to your left, or so that you are looking forward and not down toward the floor. Hold your right calf muscle with your right hand and do not let your pelvis and rib cage come unglued from your thigh, *79k.* You do not need to straighten your leg to experience stretch; you need to keep your upper body glued to your thigh and have your weight in front of your right sitz bone in order to have this position provide you with an effective stretch. Hold this position for 30 seconds to a minute. **(3)** Now turn your upper body to face down toward your leg in the same way you did in step 1, and in addition try to turn your body to see behind yourself. Keep your upper body glued to your thigh. Try to put your head down on the floor behind your right leg, *79l.* This is, of course, impossible, but by trying to put your body into this position you will be stretching some little muscles that the other positions have not yet sufficiently stretched. Hold this position for 30 seconds to a minute. **(4)** Move your upper body just in front of your right leg and hold your right foot with your right hand so you can help yourself pull down. Reach your left arm forward on the floor and put your hand down as far away from your body as you can reach. Now pull your upper body

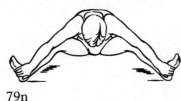

79n

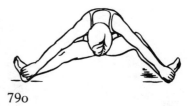

79o

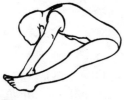

79p

down and try to touch the top of your head to the floor right in front of your right leg, *79m.* Your upper body is reaching to the right on a diagonal along the line of your right leg. Hold this position for 30 seconds to a minute. Repeat steps 1–4 on your left side.

When you have completed this sequence of stretch positions on both sides, you are ready to try to touch your head to the floor in the middle between your legs.

STARTING POSITION: With your legs spread wide apart, bend both of your legs. Bend your upper body forward at your hip sockets and put your hands on the inside of your arches or hold on to your ankles, *79n.*

THE STRETCH: Pull your upper body down to the floor as far as you can by bending your elbows. Keep your upper body in this low position and slowly extend first your right leg a little and then your left a little. *79o.* Repeat the process of extending each leg a little, one at a time, until you are as low as you can be. Now bend your elbows and pull your head down farther to touch the floor, if your head is not already on the floor, *79p.* Hold this position for 30 seconds to a minute. {**Troubleshooting:** For this process to work, you need to do this stretch in this sequence. If you straighten your legs and then pull your upper body, your pelvis is at the wrong angle to allow you to achieve maximum stretch and you will risk hurting your back.}

When you finish this stretch, you should do the Pretzel (exercise 56). In order to achieve even greater inner thigh stretch, you need to be able to open your legs wider apart. That will happen after you do the next outer thigh strengthening exercise, Doggie at the Hydrant (exercise 80).

80   DOGGIE AT THE HYDRANT

STARTING POSITION: Kneel on all fours on the floor. Place your hands directly under your shoulders. Hold in your abdominal muscles, align your head, with your chin in, and untuck your feet so that the tops are flat on the floor. Lift your bent right leg and bring your knee very close to your right armpit. Make sure that your bent leg is parallel to the floor. Check that your knee is not drooping down or pointing up. When you have lifted your leg to begin this exercise, your weight shifts to your left. *80a.*

THE STRENGTHENING EXERCISE: **(1)** Extend your lower leg and hold this position 2 counts. Make sure that your knee is pointing forward, neither up nor down, *80b.* **(2)** Lift your entire leg up 1 to 2 inches and hold this new position for 2 counts. **(3)** Move your entire right leg forward 1 to 2 inches, *80c,* and hold this position for 2 counts. **(4–5, 6–7)** Repeat steps 2 and 3 twice more: lift up, *80d,* hold 2 counts; move forward, hold 2 counts. **(8)** Hold your last position for 2 counts. Carefully bring your right leg down and repeat this exercise with your left leg. When you finish this exercise, go back to the last step in the Final Straddle part of the Three-Part Straddle Stretch (exercise 79). Follow the instructions carefully, and when you have pulled your upper body down after extending each of your legs, then gently push each leg farther out to each side. You will be able to spread your legs apart 2 to 4 inches farther to each side. Then pull your upper body down farther than it was before you pushed your legs more to each side. Hold this low position for 30 seconds to a minute.

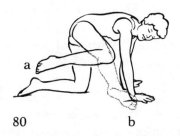

80   b

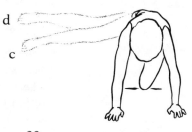

80

81 STRENGTHENING FROM STRADDLE STRETCH

You can strengthen your inner thigh muscles in this stretched position and thereby train these leg muscles to be able to hold your legs open when you are in any other position, such as standing, leaping, or running hurdles.

STARTING POSITION: Remain in the lowest stretched position of the sitting part of the Three-Part Straddle Stretch (exercise 79). Hold in your abdominal muscles. Deliberately bend your knees and feel the bottoms of your heels press on the floor.

THE STRENGTHENING EXERCISE: (1) Lift up your head so it is extended straight out from your neck. Don't grit your teeth. (2) Lift up your arms from this position of holding on to your feet, and extend them out just above your legs. (3) Slowly lift your upper body up to come to a vertical sitting position. Take 4 counts to do this. {**Troubleshooting:** This is very difficult. Be careful to hold in your abdominal muscles; don't push out on them. To hold the weight of your upper body, press down on your heels, not on locked knees.} (4) Lower your extended (not rounded) upper body down almost to the floor. Take 4 counts to do this. (5) Again lift up your upper body to a sitting position, taking 4 counts. When you finish this sequence, be sure to do the Pretzel (exercise 56).

82 PARENTHESES

This exercise trains your outer thigh muscles to guide your knees directly over your feet when you stand and walk. It is primarily to teach you to feel where your outward rotators are so you can then use them when you are doing other activities.

STARTING POSITION: Stand with your feet 4 to 6 inches apart so that your legs are straight down from their hip sockets. Align your upper body, with your abdominal muscles held in and your chin in. Bend your knees as though you are going to sit. Make sure that your knees are directly over your feet. Keep your entire foot on the floor; that is, don't bend your knees so low that you lift your heels off the floor. Press your toes, especially your big toes. Pressing your toes will help you keep the entire surface of your feet on the floor throughout this exercise.

THE STRENGTHENING EXERCISE: **(1)** Open your knees as though you were drawing parentheses in front of you with your knees, *82*. Feel the muscles on the outside of your thighs do this movement. Take 4 counts to do this. *Do not let any part of your feet move!* The entire surface of your foot remains on the floor. This is a small movement: your knees move only about 2 to 3 inches. **(2)** Hold this open position for 4 counts. **(3)** Allow your knees to return to the starting position, with your knees directly over your feet. Repeat this exercise 5 to 6 more times. {**Troubleshooting:** If you feel any pain or discomfort in your knees, you may have opened your knees too far or you may have distributed your weight too far forward on your feet. Or you may have not bent your legs enough to start with. Adjust this exercise to eliminate any knee discomfort whatsoever. You should not feel any sensation in your knee joints.}

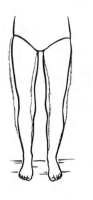

82

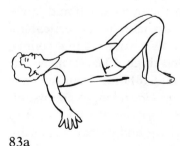

83a

83

LEG EXTENSIONS FROM HIP CURL

In Chapter 9 the Hip Curl (exercise 58) is described as a four-part sequence. You can add the following leg movements when you are in the last lifted position, with 1 or 2 ribs lifted off the floor. These leg extensions strengthen both your inner and outer thigh muscles. You will feel the front and the back of your thighs working also.

STARTING POSITION: Lie on your back on the floor or bed. Bend your knees and put your feet very near your buttocks, *83a*. Lengthen your neck, relax your jaw, and place your arms out to your sides at shoulder height, palms up. As you do this exercise, press your toes so that you distribute your weight evenly on your feet. This will prevent your hamstrings from cramping. Tighten your buttocks muscles, then lift your pelvis, your waistline, and 1 or 2 of your ribs. Now you must move your left foot 2 to 3 inches to the right to

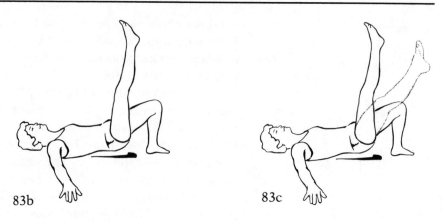

83b

83c

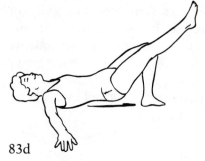

83d

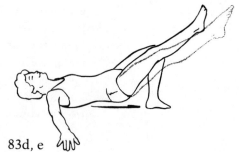

83d, e

hold your weight so you can lift up your right leg and hold it parallel to your left thigh.

THE STRENGTHENING EXERCISE: **(1)** Lift your right leg up so it is vertical, *83b*. Take 4 counts to do this. **(2)** Open it out to the right, *83c,* in 4 counts. **(3)** Lift it back up to the vertical position in 4 counts. **(4)** Cross your leg to the left in 4 counts and feel this stretch in the outer thigh and lower gluteal muscles. **(5)** Lift your leg up again to its vertical position, *83b,* taking 4 counts. **(6)** Lower your leg in 4 counts, so it is again parallel with your left thigh, *83d.* **(7)** Open your leg out to the right, *83e,* in 4 counts. **(8)** Close your leg back to the starting extended position, *83d,* taking 4 counts. **(9)** Bend your knee and put your right foot on the floor next to your left so you can lift your left leg and repeat this entire sequence with your left leg. You can rearrange the order in which you do these steps. For instance, you can start with steps 7 and 8 and then do steps 3, 4, and 5. You can also make one wide circle in either direction, as long as you do each part slowly. You will feel each muscle group working as you do this exercise. {**Troubleshooting:** To prevent your hamstrings from cramping, make sure that your feet are very close to your buttocks. Press down all the toes of your supporting foot. When you are lifting and lowering your moving leg, make sure to hold your upper body and pelvis still. Don't let the hip of your moving leg drop down or lift up. Keep it in the same place as if you had two feet on the floor.}

XIII-A

13 Your Lower Leg

Anatomy

Your lower leg consists of two bones that connect your knee to your ankle and foot *(XIII-A)*. The tibia is the thick bone that connects directly to the femur at your knee and to the talus bone in your ankle. The fibula is the narrow bone situated just to the outside of the tibia. These two lower leg bones allow your foot to rotate in a way similar to the way your forearm bones (radius and ulna) allow your hand to rotate. Ligaments securely connect these two bones in their joints and in their proper position in relationship to each other.

Your entire leg moves by means of three joints: the hip joint, the knee joint, and the ankle joint. Most of the time, when you move any part of your leg, you need to move at more than one joint. These movements are automatic; you rarely think about them unless one hurts, or you are learning new ways to move.

So your lower leg moves when you bend your knee, and, when weight bearing, when you move your ankle. Your tibia and fibula move backward at the knee from a straight line, and forward again into your legs' extended position. When your foot is off the floor, you can move your foot to each side and feel your tibia and fibula turn in relationship to each

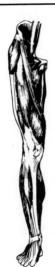

XIII-B

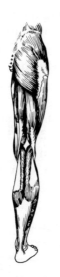

XIII-C

other the way a dancing couple revolves on the dance floor and maintains its spatial unity. These bones don't rotate around each other the way your forearm bones do.

The muscles of your lower leg help to move your leg at your knee and also control most of the parts of your foot *(XIII-B, XIII-C)*. (This chapter focuses on how your lower leg muscles enable your knee and ankle to move. The next chapter, "Your Feet," will complete the picture by telling you how your ankle and toes work.) From sad experience, you may know that the very front of your shin bone is not covered by muscles. But you do have four muscles that attach on the front sides of your two leg bones. These move the top of your foot up into a flexed position, and two of these muscles also extend your toes. You have five muscles on the back part of your lower leg. The biggest two, the gastrocnemius and soleus are your calf muscles. They both insert in the Achilles tendon at the back of your heel. They produce the opposite action from the muscles in the front of your lower leg bones: they extend your foot at the ankle, and two of them help flex your toes. These are the muscles that are so busy when you walk or run. There are two muscles on the outside of your lower leg that assist your calf muscles in extending your foot. They also let you move your foot sideways, toward the little-toe side of your leg, and turn your foot over so your big toe is on the ground and your little toe is up in the air. (See Sand Scraping [exercise 92] in the next chapter.)

Because of the way your foot extensors — the calf muscles — work when you stand, walk, jump, and run, they need a lot of stretching. Only if injured do they need much strengthening. Yet you probably have a strong and less-strong leg, so your weaker calf muscle may need strengthening to make its control similar to the stronger one. The front and side muscles of your lower leg will get stretched and strengthened doing the ankle and toe exercises in Chapter 14.

See Chapter 16 for ways to care for sore knees, pain behind the knee, and sore Achilles tendon.

Exercises

84   SITTING CALF STRETCH

STARTING POSITION: Sit on the floor with both of your legs straight in front of you and both knees bent. You will stretch one calf muscle and then the other, so relax the leg you are not stretching. Rock your upper body forward so you are folded at your hip sockets. Hold in your abdominal muscles and extend your neck straight out, with your chin in. Put your right forearm under your right knee to keep your leg from straightening out, because you may not have stretched your hamstrings, the muscles in back of your thighs.

THE STRETCH: Reach forward with your left arm so you can take your right foot in your hand. Put your left hand around the inside of your foot at your main arch and under the ball of your foot. Now gently pull your foot back; that is, flex your ankle with your hand, *84a.* Hold this stretch for 30 seconds to a minute. Be sure to keep your heel on the floor and relax your toes. Do not bend your toes back with your hand, but flex your entire foot with your hand holding on at the ball of your foot. Repeat this stretch on your left leg by putting your left arm under your left knee and using your right hand to pull your left foot back to stretch the calf muscles of your left leg. Hold this stretch for 30 seconds to a minute.

If you have very flexible ligaments, you may not feel this stretch unless you pick up your leg about 12 to 15 inches and hold it out at an angle to the floor, *84b.* In this case, reach with your right hand to hold the toes of your right foot.

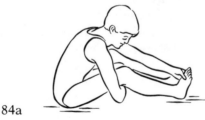

84a

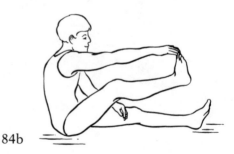

84b

Don't let your toes bend back. Gently pull your foot back and straighten your leg a little but not entirely, so you won't lock your knee and yank on your hamstrings. Keep your abdominal muscles held in and feel this stretch only in your calf muscles.

85 STANDING CALF STRETCH

STARTING POSITION: Stand and reach your right leg back about 2 to 3 feet and place it on the floor. Bend your left leg so you are in a lunge position. Lean your upper body forward so that your head, chest, and abdominal area are in a long diagonal line. Feel the weight of your body over your bent left leg. Keep your left foot flat, heel down. Take care to place your right foot straight back so your heel is directly behind your toes. Don't turn your foot out or in.

THE STRETCH: By simply standing in this position and pressing your heel down, *85*, you should be feeling a strong stretch sensation in your right calf muscle. Hold this position for 30 seconds or so.

Now relax your right knee, even if your right heel comes off the floor a half inch. By relaxing your knee, you should feel the stretch move lower or higher in your calf muscles. Remember, you have two very strong muscles on the outer surface and others underneath. Hold this stretch for 30 seconds to a minute. In order to increase the stretch, place your extended leg farther back. {**Troubleshooting:** You should not feel any sensation at all directly behind your knee. If you do, then you have received an important signal that your calf muscles are excessively tight and you need the corrective Phone Book stretch (exercise 88). If you don't feel any stretch sensation, press your pelvis forward.} Repeat this stretch on the other leg by reaching your left leg back and bending your right knee. Hold this stretch for 30 seconds to a minute. Make sure to hold the stretch on the leg that feels tighter, since everyone has a stronger leg and the muscles in your stronger leg are usually tighter.

Once you actually know the feel of the stretch in your calf muscles, then you can lean against the wall if you need to for balance (exercise 86).

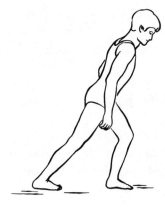

85

86

WALL CALF STRETCH

STARTING POSITION: Stand about a foot and a half away from a wall. Reach your right leg back 2 to 3 feet from your supporting leg. Make sure that your stretching foot is straight back, with your heel directly behind your toes. You must be far enough away from the wall to feel the stretch in your calf muscles, so if necessary, move your supporting leg farther back from the wall. The most important thing to remember is to lean on the wall. Do not push back from it or you will stop feeling any stretch sensation in your calf muscles.

THE STRETCH: By simply standing in this position and pressing your heel down, you should be feeling a strong stretch sensation in your calf muscles. Hold the stretch for 30 seconds to a minute. If you don't feel any stretch it may be because your upper body is forward but your pelvis is not. Press your pelvis forward so that your entire body is in one long diagonal line from your heel to your head. Remember to hold in your abdominal muscles, and do not allow your back to arch.

Now relax your knee and feel the stretch travel higher or lower in your calf muscles. Hold this position for 30 seconds to a minute.

Repeat this stretch on your other leg. Don't stretch both legs at the same time, even against the wall, because each of your legs is different in strength and flexibility. You will be better able to feel the tightness relax when you stretch one leg at a time.

87

A-FRAME CALF STRETCH

Once you have completed the sitting and standing calf stretches, you are ready for this next position. This one is very strong, so you need to ready your muscles with the first two stretches.

STARTING POSITION: From the lunge position of the Standing Calf Stretch (exercise 85), bend down and put both of your hands on the floor, 2 to 3 feet in front of your back leg, which may be your left leg since that is the one you just

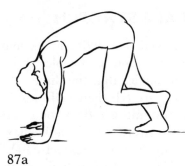

87a

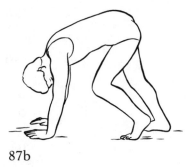

87b

finished stretching. Now bring your right foot back and rest the front of your right foot on the back of your left ankle, *87a*. If this position produces too strong a stretch, then, with your right leg bent, put your right foot down on the floor about 6 to 8 inches forward of your left foot. Rest the ball of that foot down so it can bear a little weight, *87b*.

THE STRETCH: Just by getting into this position, *87a*, you will feel this strong stretch in the weight-bearing left ankle. Your body weight is causing the tractionlike pull against your calf muscles. Relax your knee. If your left heel comes off the floor slightly, that is okay. In fact, in this position, it is very hard to keep your heel on the floor. If it is not a strong stretch for you, widen your A-frame by moving your hands forward 6 to 12 inches. If it is too strong, narrow the A-frame by moving your hands closer to your feet until you can tolerate the strong stretch sensation. Keep your left heel on or very near the floor. Hold this stretch for 30 seconds to a minute. Repeat this stretch on your right leg. Hold the stretch longer on your tighter leg. Most people are unevenly strong, and so one leg always needs more time to stretch and the other often needs less.

88   PHONE BOOK CALF STRETCH

This stretch is an orthopedic corrective for people with excessively tight calf muscles and for people who have such loose ligaments in their ankles that the three calf stretches above do not adequately stretch their calf muscles. If your body fits one of these descriptions, then you should do this stretch. Before doing this stretch, do the ankle flexibility exercise in Chapter 14, Foot Crisscross (exercise 91).

STARTING POSITION: Put a 2- to 3-inch phone book on the floor about a foot from a wall. Have the pages closest to you and the binding near the wall. Now slide the pages into a wedge shape. This wedge helps pull on your calf muscles from a second direction, from below, whereas the regular calf stretch only pulls on your calf muscles from one direction, above. Put your right foot on the wedged pages so that the ball of your foot is all the way on the cover. Put your other foot next to the phone book on the floor. You will stretch one calf muscle at a time. Press the toes of your right foot gently on the phone book.

THE STRETCH: (1) Lean your upper body forward and rest your bent arms on the wall in front of you, *88a*. You should feel the stretch very strongly in your right calf. If you don't, then make sure that your pelvis is forward and that you are not bending only from your waist. Your leaning position must have your entire body in a long diagonal line toward the wall from your heel up to your head. If you still don't

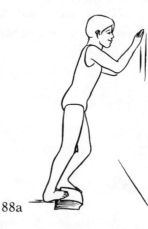

88a   88b

feel the stretch very strongly in your calf, then move the phone book farther away from the wall, about 4 to 6 inches. If the stretch is too strong, open the phone book to take away 1 inch of its height. Hold the stretch as long as you can tolerate the stretch sensation. That means only holding the position for 30 seconds to a minute on the first day. Only hold it as long as you are comfortable doing so, because the stretch is strong. **(2)** Bend your right knee a little and this will move the stretch sensation higher or lower in those two muscles and allow you to remain longer in the stretch position, *88b.*

Now change legs. Put your left foot on the wedge-shaped phone book and put your right foot on the floor next to the phone book. Lean against the wall. Hold the stretch position as long as you are comfortable doing so.

Each day you will lengthen the time you can hold this stretch position. Your goal, believe it or not, is to work up to 5 minutes a day on each leg. That may take six weeks, but you must work up to this length of time gradually. {**Troubleshooting:** Don't do this stretch on a step: it is too easy to slip because your heel has no support. Don't do it on a square book, either, because the sharp corner pushes into your arch and can make your foot uncomfortable. Especially, do not rise up onto the ball of your foot and then let your heel sink down to the floor over and over, as some exercise programs instruct you to do. With extra-tight calf muscles, this severe contraction followed by a severe stretch can trigger the circuit breakers in your tendon and then you risk rupturing it.}

After doing this stretch you should be able to do the Standing Calf Stretch and the A-frame Calf Stretch (exercises 85, 87) and feel the stretch sensations. So if you need this corrective stretch, then do it first, and then do the other two standing stretches.

89

ONE-FOOTED HEEL RAISES

This exercise helps strengthen your calf muscles. It is especially effective after an injury or prolonged immobility, such as having your foot or leg in a cast. You can also use it simply to remedy the uneven strength of your legs.

STARTING POSITION: Stand near a wall or ledge so you can hold on to something for balance. Place your feet straight forward, and now lift your right leg up by bending your knee. You will hold your right leg in this position while you strengthen your left leg.

THE STRENGTHENING EXERCISE: **(1)** Slowly bend your left knee, taking 2 counts. **(2)** Now rise up on the ball of your foot and straighten but do not lock your knee at the same time, *89*. Take two counts to do this. **(3)** Now bend your knee and replace your heel on the floor in 2 counts. This is almost a slow motion hop. Continue this slow rise-and-straighten, bend-and-lower action as long as you can. Your goal is to be able to repeat this thirty times. Keep your knee aligned above your foot, so it does not lean out or in. Your upper thigh — your quadriceps muscles — will share the benefit and get very tired and strong doing this exercise. Repeat the exercise on the other leg. Be sure to stretch your calf and upper thigh muscles before and after doing this strenuous strengthening exercise.

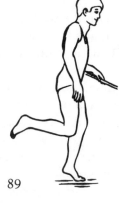

89

90

SLOW MOTION JUMPING

Jumping is especially good for building strong leg muscles.

STARTING POSITION: Stand with your feet about 6 inches apart and facing forward. Don't hold on to anything while you do this exercise. Align your head above your rib cage, hold in your abdominal muscles, and make sure to breathe evenly.

THE STRENGTHENING EXERCISE: **(1)** Bend your knees, *90a*. **(2)** Try jumping slowly ten times, *90b*. You do this with two feet, using the same movements you used for One-Footed Heel Raises (exercise 89). You will not be able to stay in the air for two counts, but jump as slowly as you can. Feel

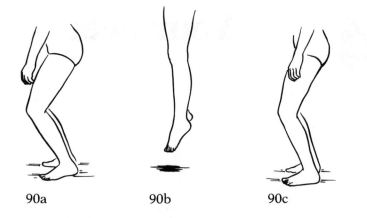

90a   90b   90c

your calf muscles do the work. Make sure to let your heels come completely down on the ground with each landing, *90c*. When you speed up, you will then get help from all your other leg muscles, and they help you anyway. You can do slow hops, on one leg and then on the other, and get the same strengthening result. {**Troubleshooting:** Make sure you bend your knees each time your feet come down to the ground and align your knees above your feet. You should also press down your toes when doing this strengthening exercise. A lot more will be said about your toes in Chapter 14.}

Note: To take proper care of your knees, you need to keep your knees unlocked. See Alignment (exercise 98) in Chapter 15 and the sections on sore knees, sore back, and pain in the groin in Chapter 16. Also have your legs measured. If one leg is shorter, then wear a heel lift, usually only ¼ to ⅜ of an inch high, under that heel. See Chapter 16.

14 Your Feet

Anatomy

Have you ever thought about how much your feet do for you? They are relatively small compared to the rest of your body, yet they hold all of you up, they are your base of support; and they propel you in any direction you choose. They push you off the ground and receive all of your weight on them when you land. Three cheers for your feet! They are structured to provide your body both a stable and a mobile base.

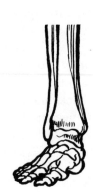

XIV-A

Each of your feet has 26 bones, one less than each of your hands. Your ankle has seven bones; your mid-foot, where your long arch is, has five long bones; and your toes, like your fingers, have three bones each and your big toe has two. All these bones are securely bound together with many ligaments, and these ligaments are more responsible for the stability of your foot than your muscles are. The tibia rests on top of the talus bone, which is on top of the calcaneus bone. This lowest bone in the stack is your heel bone, to which the Achilles tendon is attached. The bumps on the sides of your ankle are the sides of the bottom ends of the tibia on the inside and the fibula on the outside. The other four ankle bones are smaller and in front of the two big ankle bones *(XIV-A)*.

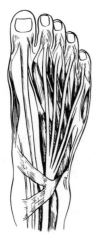

XIV-B

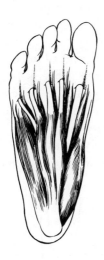

XIV-C

At your ankle joints, your feet have a similar range of motion as your hands do at your wrists. When you are not standing on them, they can move up so that your toes come closer to your lower legs; down so your feet are pointed and your ankles and feet make almost a straight line; to each side; and around in circles. Your toes can curl up and down, spread apart, and close. With great concentration, you can get each toe to move in a circle *(XIV-B and C)*.

You have two arches in each foot. The main one is the longitudinal arch. This is what you mean when you worry about your arch falling. It curves off the floor on the inside, the big-toe side, of your foot. Your other arch runs across your foot, under the ball of your foot where your long mid-foot bones meet the shorter bones of your toes. Both your arches provide spring action for your feet and, though their shape is chiefly maintained by ligaments, you can protect them and nurture them if you strengthen and use your toes in the way they are meant to be used. The Inchworm (exercise 95) specifically strengthens the muscles of these arches.

You can see that, with so many bones in your feet, if you use your feet off-center or out of alignment, you will rearrange the bones while they are carrying you around. This misplaced weight can stretch the ligaments that bind your foot bones together, and these ligaments don't unstretch. Then you could lose some of the built-in springiness of your feet. So it really pays to use your feet correctly, by stepping on them straight forward and pressing down with your toes. (You will read more about this process in Chapter 15, "Putting It All Together.") In this chapter you will learn exercises to help you use your feet correctly so they can continue to do their basic (pun intended!) job for you and your body.

Your ankle is similar to your wrist in that the exercises that strengthen one side of it will stretch the other side at the same time. The exercises for your toes will also contribute to the strength and stability of your ankle, so keep that in mind when you are working on your ankle.

Chapter 16 describes how to take care of fallen arches, sore toes, and sore feet.

Exercises

91 ANKLE CRISSCROSS

This exercise helps your ankle bend more completely than it does after doing two or three calf stretches. Be sure to do this before you do any leg activity.

STARTING POSITION: You can do this exercise sitting or standing. It is important that your lower leg be straight down and your ankle extended, with your toes pointing down, *91a.*

When you are standing, hold on to something for balance and bend your right knee and lift your foot off the floor 4 to 6 inches. When sitting, you can hold your thigh up a little off the chair, with your knee bent so your lower leg is pointing straight down. The hard part of the exercise is that you need to relax your toes and not use them when you lift or lower your foot. So, to give your toes something to do, use your toe muscles to keep your toes together and extended. Don't curl them up or under.

THE EXERCISE: **(1)** Slowly lift your right foot up toward your lower leg, *91a,* taking 4 counts. This is sometimes called flexing your foot. Don't use your toes when you do this. **(2)** Slowly extend your foot to point down to the floor, *91a,* in 4 counts. As you do this, pretend you are pressing something under your foot. **(3)** Slowly press your foot in to your left, *91c,* taking 4 counts. Pretend your foot is the pen-

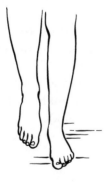

91a   91b   91a

dulum of a clock. Don't move it so far to the side that it starts to come into a flexed position. Your foot won't move very far to the side. **(4)** Now move your foot back down to your starting position, *91a*, taking 4 counts. **(5)** Now move it sideways to the right, *91d*, in 4 counts. **(6)** Move your foot back to your starting position, *91a*, in 4 counts. Repeat this sequence, going up, down, side, and side, one more time. **(7)** Now you are going to draw a circle to the right with your foot and take 10 to 12 counts to do it. Don't use your toes. **(8)** Finally, draw that circle going around the other way, to the left. Take 10 to 12 counts to do this. Repeat this sequence on your left foot.

92

SAND SCRAPING

This exercise strengthens the muscles in your ankle that the Ankle Crisscross (exercise 91) does not. You feel this exercise on top of your foot as well as in your ankle. After you do this, you will be able to bend your ankles more than you were able to before you did the exercise. Try a before-and-after test. Here is another example of how strengthening muscles also helps them stretch more completely.

STARTING POSITION: You can do this exercise sitting or standing. Your working leg needs to be free of weight, so stand on your left leg and move your right foot forward about 4 inches. Keep the knee of your right leg relaxed or a little bent. Put your heel and the outside of your right foot on the floor, so that the big-toe side of your foot is up and the little-toe side of your foot is down, *92a*. Your arch is not touching the floor. Instead of pointing your foot straight ahead, point it diagonally to your right.

THE EXERCISE: **(1)** Pretend that you are standing on a sandy beach and that you have sand under your foot to move around. Scrape the little-toe side of your foot slowly to your left, or inward, taking 4 counts. Your foot will pivot on your heel and the toe end of your foot will make a curved pathway of about 4 inches, *92a,b*. Reach and curve your toes when you do this. **(2)** Turn your foot over so that the big-toe side of your foot is on the floor and the little-toe side is up.

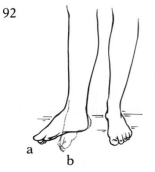

92

a   b

177

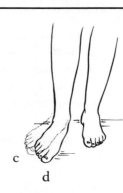

92

c

d

Your heel is still on the floor. Scrape the big-toe side of your foot to your right, or outward, as far as it will go, about 4 inches in a curved pathway, *92c,d*. **(3)** Turn your foot over so that the little-toe side is on the floor just as in step 1 and repeat this scraping motion to your left. Take 4 counts. **(4)** Repeat step 2 to your right. Repeat this exercise two more times. Make sure to curve all of your toes as though you were pushing a lot of sand. Repeat this exercise on your left foot.

93   TOE CURLS AND UNCURLS

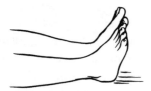

93a

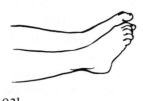

93b

These toe curls help you improve your toes' coordination at the same time that you stretch and strengthen them.

STARTING POSITION: Sit on the floor, a sofa, or a bed where you can extend your legs. Bend your knees a little and even put a small pillow under them. Rest your heels comfortably, *93a*. Sit up or rest back on your arms extended behind you. Don't lock your elbows. Hold in your abdominal muscles, and align your head, with your chin in. You will be working with both of your feet at once.

THE EXERCISE: **(1)** Curl your toes. Another way to say this is make a fist with your toes. Do the action gently and slowly so that you will not cause a cramp in your feet, *93b*. Take 4 counts to curl your toes. **(2)** Point your feet by extending your ankles, *93c*, taking 4 counts, while holding your toes in that curled position. This is hard to do; they will try to uncurl. **(3)** Flex your ankles with your toes still curled. That

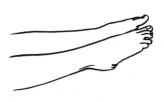

93c

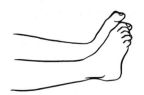

93d

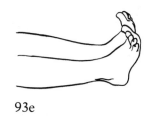

93e

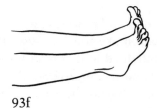

93f

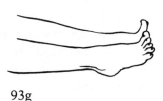

93g

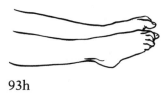

93h

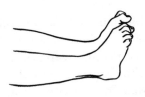

93i

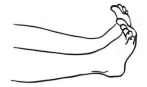

93j

means that you bend your ankles and bring your feet closer up toward your lower legs, *93d*. Take 4 counts to do this. **(4)** When your feet are as flexed as they can go and are about to change direction and extend, uncurl your toes and flex them as much as you can, *93e,f*. Do this in 4 counts. **(5)** Move your feet to their most extended position, keeping your toes flexed, *93g*. Do this in 4 counts. **(6)** When your feet are extended as far as they will go and are about to change direction, curl your toes, *93h*, in 4 counts. Repeat steps 3–6 four to six more times.

Now you will reverse this process, and curl your toes where you flexed them and flex them where you curled them. Make sure to keep your knees bent and your heels on the surface on which they are resting. **(1)** With your feet extended, pointing down, flex your toes, *93g*, in 4 counts. This is the opposite of curling them. **(2)** Flex your ankles with your toes still flexed, *93i*, in 4 counts. **(3)** Curl your toes, *93j*, taking 4 counts. **(4)** Put your feet in their most extended position, keeping your toes curled, *93h*. Do this in 4 counts. Repeat steps 1–5 and continue this sequence four to six more times.

94

TOE OPEN AND CLOSE

The purpose of this exercise is to stretch and strengthen your toe muscles. It may help get your reluctant toes to listen to directions from your brain and return to their original mobility and dexterity. This exercise can help your toes fight back against the immobilizing toe squeeze of most shoes.

STARTING POSITION: Sit where your feet can rest and your ankle can be relaxed. If your legs are extended, bend your knees or even put a small pillow under them. Align the rest of your body.

THE EXERCISE: **(1)** Extend your toes and at the same time spread them apart as far as you can make them go, *94*. Do this in 4 counts. **(2)** Hold them extended and spread for 4 counts. **(3)** Close your toes together and still try to keep them extended, stretched out, in 4 counts. Repeat this open-and-close, spread-and-squeeze sequence six to ten times, or as much as you have patience for. At first, exercising your toes may be frustrating because you may not be accustomed to coordinating that area of your body. Be patient with yourself and keep working; you will get very beneficial results. A more difficult way to do this exercise is to point your foot and then try to spread, extend, and hold your toes apart. Good luck!

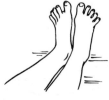

94

95

INCHWORM

This is one of the most important exercises you can do for your feet. The Inchworm strengthens your metatarsal arch and toe muscles. This exercise gives your toes the strength they need to press down every time you stand, walk, run, or jump on your feet. With this strength, you will be able to balance, stand, walk, and run with more power, control, and stability. You can do it anytime you have an empty moment. It is well worth the time and effort.

STARTING POSITION: This exercise can be done sitting or standing. You will be working with one foot at a time. If you are standing, unlock your left leg, which will support you while you exercise your right foot. Point your feet straight

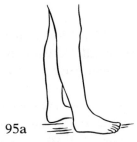
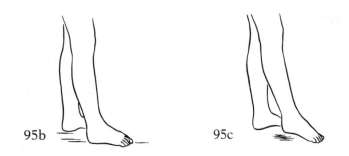

95a   95b   95c

ahead. Align the rest of your body in the same way that you have for all the other exercises. If you are sitting, bend your knees so your lower legs are straight down and both your feet are on the floor. It is best to do this exercise barefoot. *95a.*

THE STRENGTHENING EXERCISE: **(1)** Press the bottoms of all five of your toes down on the floor and lift up the entire ball of your foot, *95b*. This action should pull your heel closer to your toes and arch up your entire foot. {**Trouble-shooting:** The action of your toes pressing down is *not* curling them. The action is more like pressing your feet into sand or clay to make an imprint.} Press your toes firmly and pull your heel toward your toes in 4 counts. **(2)** Now reach your toes forward, not up, and rest your toes and the ball of your foot back down on the floor in 4 counts. Repeat this inching forward five more times. **(3)** To bring your foot back to be next to your other one, press your toes, lift the entire ball of your foot, and lift your heel off the floor about 1 to 2 inches and firmly pull your foot, leading with your heel, back to be next to your left foot, *95c*. Take 4 to 6 counts to do this. When you do this action, you should feel the contraction of the muscles under the ball of your foot, in your metatarsal area. The Inchworm strengthens the stretched muscles in that arch. {**Troubleshooting:** The shape of your foot as you lift up the ball of your foot is a gentle curve toward your toes. If you do not have your arch lifted enough, the shape of your foot above the ball of your foot will be flat. That happens when you curl your toes and allow them to tuck under instead of press down.}

Repeat the Inchworm once more on your right foot and then do it twice on your left foot.

96

HEEL RAISES

This exercise is described as One-Footed Heel Raises (exercise 89) in Chapter 13 to strengthen your calf. Here are more specific instructions about how you should use your toes when you do that exercise.

STARTING POSITION: Assume the same position as for One-Footed Heel Raises. You can use one foot or both feet, and you can hold on to something for balance if you need to. Be sure to keep your knees unlocked.

THE EXERCISE: (1) Slowly bend your knees, taking 2 counts. Make sure that your knees are aligned directly over your feet and not inside or outside them. **(2)** Now rise up on the balls of your feet and straighten (but do not lock) your knees at the same time. Do this in 2 counts. **(3)** Bend your knees and replace your heels on the floor, taking 2 counts. As you lift your heels, press your toes down and keep them pressing. Only lift your heels as high as you can and still feel the weight of your body on the entire ball of your foot, *96*. {**Troubleshooting:** If you lift your heels too high, your toes will no longer be able to press down and you will move forward to the front of the ball of your foot. Going too high onto the front of the ball of your foot actually stretches your metatarsal arch muscles and this weakens your foot.} As you bend your knees and lower your heels to the floor, keep pressing your toes. You will have much more control of your balance when you use your toes this way. This is true for your feet whether you are walking, running, skiing, or ice-skating. In other words, whenever you press down your toes, you will be strengthening your toes, protecting your foot and ankle, and preventing knee injury.

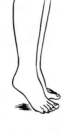

96

97

HICCUP

This is a challenging toe and foot strengthening exercise that helps you jump and land using your toe muscles. If your toes are passive when you take off and land from a jump or a leap (each running step is a small leap), you stretch your metatarsal arch and weaken your entire foot.

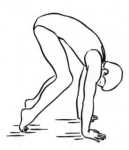

97a

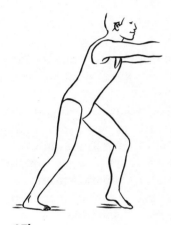

97b

Before beginning this exercise, you should bend down, put both of your hands on the floor, and rock your weight forward so you can lift yourself up onto the tips of your toes, *97a*. Doing this will let you feel in your toes the effort they will be making when doing this exercise.

STARTING POSITION: Assume the same position as for the Standing Calf Stretch (exercise 85). Place your right leg back about 3 feet from your left leg. Bend the knee of your left leg. Lean your upper body diagonally forward so the weight of your body is over your bent left leg. Hold in your abdominal muscles and align your head, with your chin in. Reach your arms forward. Lift your left heel about 3 inches. *97b*.

THE STRENGTHENING EXERCISE: (1) Using only your toes, try to lift your left knee up toward your face. Your effort will be to lift all of the weight that is on your left foot by contracting your toes and starting to do the Inchworm (exercise 95). The direction of your left knee is up. That is the only part of your body that should move. The movement that results by doing this is small, like a hiccup. Most people cannot even lift their foot off the floor an inch. {**Troubleshooting:** If you do lift up your foot more than that, then you will have pushed your weight back onto your back leg enough to have your front thigh muscles lift your leg, and your body will have moved back, not up.} Repeat this exercise four to eight times. Before you repeat this with your right leg forward, make sure to take time to stretch your left calf muscle, because it stays in a contracted state while you are doing the Hiccup.

You may have to practice the Inchworm and the Hiccup for a few weeks before they will work for you.

15 Putting It All Together

This book is about your body. And this chapter should come first, but if it were first you would not know what you now know about your body.

Stand up and close your eyes. Feel your feet being pulled to the floor by the force of gravity and experience your entire body extending up into the universe. (Take a minute to do this.) If you are like most people, you don't take the time to experience your entire body as an entity separate from your thoughts, your self-image, positive and negative, or the separate parts of your body that you like or don't like.

This book has led you through a series of exercises for each major part of your body. The readying and starting positions for each section and each exercise told you where to put all your body parts. The more you are aware of one part in relation to another, the more you will sense your entire physical wholeness. And the more flexible and strong the muscles for each of your parts are, the more easily you will sense, control, and enjoy your body. That is your goal, isn't it?

The topics in this chapter are for your whole body. In breathing, alignment, balance, walking, running, and jumping, you experience yourself as a whole, as an entity. Enjoy!

*

Breathing

DO IT! The cardinal rule about breathing is, Keep it up. Don't stop! Whether it is chest breathing, or stomach breathing, or deep breathing, or shallow breathing, it doesn't matter as long as you are breathing. As a matter of fact, there is a lot of contradictory information about the subject. When you experiment with the various breathing instructions, judge their effectiveness by how you feel doing them. You may not breathe deeply enough, but you can't really breathe the "wrong" way.

Recent research shows that your lungs expand in response to your physical activity. That is good news because you know that your lungs are taking care of themselves as you go about your business. The only thing you need to pay attention to is whether your breathing mechanism is functioning freely. That means noticing what state your breathing is in and being sure not to hold your breath.

Making sure you're not holding your breath is very important. When doing some of the strengthening exercises in this book, you may find yourself almost holding your breath because they are, at first, so strenuous. For instance, when you do Curl-downs (exercise 47), you may have to breathe in and hold your breath for 10 seconds in order to hold in your middle abdominal muscle. Instead of actually holding your breath, try counting out loud. This will cause you to do superficial breathing and still allow you to hold in your abdominal muscle. If you can't count out loud, and if you really do hold your breath, it probably won't hurt you to do so for 6 to 10 seconds. You hold your breath for longer than that when you swim under water. In no other exercise in this book will there be a need for you to hold your breath. If you do, then you are working with too much intensity and need to relax a little.

Paying attention to your breathing is much harder than it would appear at first. Most people are oblivious to their breathing because it is so automatic. It speeds up when you are excited; it slows down as you relax; it adjusts to the loudness or softness of your voice. It comes with more difficulty when you are scared. Often these changes in breathing go unnoticed. By checking in on the state of your breathing as you go about your daily activities, you will get a lot of good information. Whatever you learn, use that information to guide yourself. Remember the rule of thumb: Keep breathing.

Regular deep breathing can relax your body and lessen stress. Barbara B. Brown, in her book *Between Health and Illness* (Boston: Houghton Mifflin, 1984), suggests that the practice of regular deep breathing can prevent the stress in your life from wearing down your immune system and thereby keep you from getting many diseases. *Relaxation Response* (New York: Avon, 1976), by Herbert Benson and Miriam C. Klipper, describes the same phenomenon. While you are exercising, you need to pay attention first to the stretching or strengthening sensations in your muscles and not have any unpleasant or uncomfortable feeling in your joints. Then you need to notice how your breathing is going and make sure that it is going on steadily.

If you practice regular deep breathing while you are stretching your muscles, you may find that your muscles relax more easily while stretching. If you deliberately breathe on every other count of the strengthening exercises, then you may find that the exercises feel more comfortable. Research has also shown that you will feel less fatigue in your muscles if you maintain a steady breathing pattern. So not only is regular and free breathing good for preventing stress, it also helps you achieve the results you want from these exercises.

Exercises

98   ALIGNMENT

Your body is a single unit, a whole entity. However, the chapters in this book have discussed each major part of your body separately. To compensate for this way of organizing the exercises, throughout the *readying positions* and the *starting positions* you have been instructed to align the parts of your body above and below the part you are exercising.

This must have provided you a strong clue that your parts are all connected, just as the old song says: Your foot bone's connected to your ankle bone. Your ankle bone's connected to your leg bone. And so forth all the way up the body. How well and easily your body moves depends on how ready your muscles are to move and where your body parts are located in relationship to each other. That is alignment. If your alignment is not correct, you will move inefficiently and your body parts will be more vulnerable to injury.

What is proper alignment? The guidelines for proper alignment in movement systems all over the world agree on this information. You can think about your body this way: It is made up of three hunks — your head, your rib cage, and your pelvis — suspended in front of and attached to a bendable rod, your spine. These connected hunks are supported on two long hinged rods, your legs; and your legs balance on top of two small pedestals, your feet. When these units are correctly stacked and balanced, then you will be properly aligned, *98*.

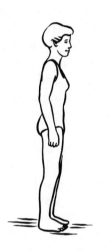

98

(1) Start at the top of your body. You head needs to be held up so that your ears are over your shoulders. In order to move your head into the correct position, lengthen your neck up. Don't lift your head from your forehead or the middle top of your head. Lift it from the back top part of your head. Just imagine that your head is the topmost bone on your spine and lift it from where your spine comes up through your skull. Get the feeling that your head is balanced on your neck, that you are not using muscles to hold it there.

(2) Now align your rib cage. Your rib cage needs to be directly above your pelvis, not leaning back or slumping forward. Inside your rib cage are your lungs. Imagine that they are air-filled balloons that suspend you in space. Then your upper body will be weightless, rather than a burden for your lower body to carry around. Your shoulders are on top of and to the side of your rib cage, and they need to be gently held down and together. Feel as though you have crisscrossing suspenders on your back pulling your shoulder blades down in diagonal lines that meet at your waistline in the shape of a diamond.

(3) Now align your pelvis. Your pelvis needs to hang down from your spine so that your back makes a relaxed vertical line. The pelvis should not be tipped back so that the natural curve at your waist increases. And it should not be tipped forward or tucked under so that you lose all of the curve in your lower back. You should use no muscular effort to keep your pelvis in proper alignment. The secret to aligning your pelvis with your rib cage correctly is to unlock your knees. When you stack your thigh bone directly above your lower leg bones in a straight line, your pelvis will naturally hang directly down in its correct vertical position. When your knees are locked (hyperextended) you unstack your leg bones, and this, in turn, tips your pelvis. This tipping back of your pelvis pulls your rib cage back, and your head, in turn, slides forward. Therefore, by unlocking your knees and stacking your leg bones one on top of the other, you can align almost all of your body correctly.

(4) Finally, align your feet. Your entire body needs to be centered over the place just behind the balls of your feet. If you stand with your knees locked, then your body weight is back on your heels and you hardly have any weight on the rest of your feet. After you unlock your knees, you need also to rock your entire body forward about an inch. This shifts your pelvis, your center of gravity, forward and makes it easier to keep your knees unlocked. This tiny forward move places your body on the entire surface of both your feet, and your toes can press the ground to hold you up, which is what they are meant to do. When you press your big toe, you will lift up your main arch and also lift your ankle. Doing this wrong by locking your knees makes your ankles fall together and you stretch the main arch in your feet. Unlocking your knees lets you balance your entire body where it belongs while also allowing you to use your feet properly.

Standing with your body correctly aligned burns the fewest possible calories. That is because proper alignment allows the muscles in the front and the back of your body to be used evenly. All your muscles work in concert to hold you up against gravity. When you stack up your body parts correctly, you help your muscles do their job in the most efficient way, the way they have been constructed to function.

99

BALANCE

When you say that you can't balance, you usually mean that you can't balance while standing on one foot. Sometimes you might feel that balance is a matter of luck. It is not luck. Here are guidelines to enable you to balance on one foot. You need to keep in mind and in your body the guidelines for correct alignment. The muscles you use to balance yourself will work more efficiently if your body parts are correctly stacked on top of each other.

GUIDELINES FOR BALANCING ON ONE FOOT: **(1)** As you stand on one leg, distribute your weight on your entire foot, pressing all five toes down as though you are making an imprint in sand or clay. **(2)** Unlock your knee. This will allow your body to remain over your entire foot. Be careful not to bend your knee; just unlock it. **(3)** Gently tighten the buttock of your standing leg and push your pelvis forward a little bit. Another way to say this is to flatten the line from the top of your thigh along the front of your pelvis. That is what happens when you tighten your buttock muscles and push your pelvis forward. **(4)** Align your head correctly above your shoulders, with your chin in.

If you follow these guidelines, you can balance anywhere, in any position, even on ice skates. The guidelines work even when your upper body is not vertical. The only one that doesn't apply is the placement of your head.

When you rise up onto the ball of your foot, you can still remain in control of your balance. You need especially to press your toes. Remember the Troubleshooting hint for Heel Raises (exercise 96): don't rise too high on your foot. When you do, your weight goes too far forward and is no longer on the entire surface of the ball of your foot, and you are no longer able to press down your toes.

100

WALKING

"Walking?" you say. "You mean I have to relearn to walk?" Walking is so natural that you don't expect that there is anything to learn. But your inherited structure, with your loose

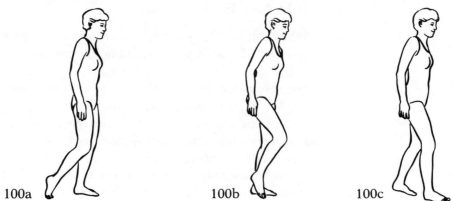

100a 100b 100c

or tight ligaments, for instance, affects whether your feet turn in or out and whether your knees lock on every step. These small mechanical problems can, over time, cause you trouble. When you walk correctly, you protect your ankles, knees, hip sockets, and lower back. When you walk with your usual little or big idiosyncrasies, you weaken, stress, or make vulnerable the joints in your legs, and this can hurt your lower back.

Here are some guidelines for correct walking. Unless your body has an unusual structure, these guidelines will help you use your body in motion in a very efficient way.

GUIDELINES FOR WALKING CORRECTLY: (1) Align your body, using the guidelines given in Alignment (exercise 98). Pay special attention to maintaining your head above your shoulders, and keep your chin in. **(2)** Keep your body weight above your front, weight-receiving foot, not over your back foot. **(3)** Aim all your moving parts straight ahead. That means your arms, which are relaxed, should swing straight ahead, not across your chest. Your knees and feet should go straight ahead, not in or out even a small bit. **(4)** Walking involves free-swinging action in your major joints. Your arms should swing freely back and forth at your shoulder. Your leg should swing freely back and forth at your hip socket. Allow your leg to swing back as far as it swings front. The Pretzel stretch (exercise 56) helps you accomplish this goal. Your bent knee swings forward and then your leg extends as your weight transfers onto it. And your ankle joint extends to push your knee forward and flexes when you place your weight on your foot. So you use your shoulder, hip, knee, and ankle joints fully on every step.

These first 4 guidelines are general ones. The next are specific for each of the moving parts in your walk. **(5)** Feel that your pelvis moves you forward on each step. By moving your pelvis forward on each step, you move your center of gravity forward. If your pelvis follows your leg movement, you essentially drag it along instead of using it to lead your walk. **(6)** Start your leg moving on every step by leading with your knee, not your foot, *100a*. Feel as though your knee goes directly forward, not up and down. **(7)** Step down on your entire foot, starting with your heel and going straight forward to your toes. **(8)** Press all of your toes each time you step down on them and each time you push off with them. The pressing down is the same as in the Inchworm (exercise 95). Don't curl your toes or lift them up excessively, and don't overbend the arch under the ball of your foot. **(9)** Shorten your usual length of step by about an inch. Small steps are more efficient because they let you maintain your alignment more easily.

There are three parts to taking a step when you walk: the push, weight transference, and weight receiving. The push happens with your back foot. To start your walk, lead with your knee. To lead with your knee you need to extend your ankle. To extend your ankle, press your toes down and lift the ball of your foot just as you do in the Inchworm. Now you are in motion.

Weight transference happens before you put your back foot down in the front of your body, *100b*. During this brief phase of the walk, your knee can wobble in and out, and that wobble can create knee pain. You need to keep pressing the toes of your front foot, which has not lifted off the floor yet.

The last part of the walk, weight receiving, happens when you put your back foot down in front of your body. Put it straight ahead, *100c*. Step on your heel and transfer your weight through your foot to your toes. Don't deliberately roll to the outside bottom edge of your foot. Your foot will receive your weight there anyway, because your main arch is on the bottom inside surface of your foot.

Your knees need special attention while you walk. At no

time during any part of the walk should your knees be locked. If you lock your knees when you stand, you are likely to lock your knee during the push part of the walk. Keep your knees relaxed and lead with each knee in turn. In this way, you can correct this harmful habit. During the weight transference, your knee is not likely to lock, but it can wobble (doing Parentheses [exercise 82] helps prevent this), so make sure to aim it straight ahead and press your toes. During the weight-receiving part of the walk, if you lead with your knee it should be bent and not locked. If you swing your straight leg forward and drop your heel down, then you will jar your knee, and that action, over time, can cause injuries. The straight-legged way of walking is very inefficient, to say the least.

When you practice walking correctly, start with one guideline at a time. For instance, lead with your knee. That action may trigger any of the others. Notice how any one action feels and see if you can feel how it differs from the way you usually walk. You need to be able to distinguish between the old habit and the new one. Then start to press your toes. Put one new guideline on "automatic pilot" before you start to implement the next one. Be patient with yourself as you correct old and probably subtle habits. Correcting your walk is well worth the effort. You are engaged in body preservation! More will be said about this subject in Chapter 16, "Special Care of Your Body."

101   RUNNING

You probably run with the same muscles and mechanical patterns that you use when you walk. So *all* the guidelines for correct walking apply when you run. Running is a series of leaps from one foot to the other. You lift your entire body off the ground and then balance on one foot for an instant as you return back down to earth from your tiny flight in space. This quality of flying makes running as popular as it is.

Your liftoff and landing need some attention. When you lift off, press your toes as in the Inchworm and Hiccup (exercises 95 and 97) and you will help your calf and buttock muscles push you up. When you land, keep two guidelines in mind and body: again, use your toes to press down; and allow all the joints in your leg to bend to absorb the impact of receiving all of your body weight. This second guideline sounds so simple, but many people don't allow it to happen. Bend! Let your thigh bend at your hip socket. Let your knee bend. Let your ankle bend as you land on your foot. And let all of your bending body parts go straight ahead, not even slightly in or out. In other words, allow your body to yield to gravity as you land. Your legs are structured to act like springs by means of your joints and muscles. When you use your legs like springs, you prevent a lot of joint injury.

If you are racing, you use what is known as "sprinter's stride," which means that you land on your toes before your heel lands. Your heel must come down to the ground to give you maximum use of all of your leg muscles. Otherwise, your calf will become so tight and inflexible that you will diminish your ability to push off. This in turn creates stress in your knees, ankles, and lower back.

When you jog, use your foot the same way that you do when you walk. That means landing with your heel first. Landing this way immediately moves your weight forward onto the entire surface of your foot. Take small steps, just as in walking, to keep your entire upper body over your front, weight-receiving foot. Make sure that your head is aligned and your chin is in.

102

JUMPING

All you need to know about jumping has been said in the sections on alignment, balance, walking, and running. When you are jumping in a vertical posture, then proper alignment allows you to jump most efficiently. Most jumps, however, are not done in a vertical posture, so the alignment guidelines can be helpful only some of the time.

GUIDELINES FOR JUMPING: (1) Use the spring action of your leg joints and muscles. (2) Make sure to land onto the entire surface of your foot, which means letting your heel go

193

down to the ground. **(3)** Press your toes to lift off and to land. The pressing action is the same as in the Inchworm (exercise 95), where you try to lift the ball of your foot up. **(4)** Make sure that your knees bend directly over your feet and not in or out. To check this, bend your knees, jump, and land. Keep your body in the final position of your landing and look straight down over your knees to see if your feet are directly below your knees. Practice jumping and landing with your heels coming down to the ground and your knees bending directly over your feet. This is not easy to do, but it is very worthwhile. You are again engaged in body preservation.

16 Special Care of Your Body

This chapter will help you deal with special problems and recover from injury. The information here in no way replaces diagnosis and treatment by a physician. There are two kinds of injuries: very severe and not so severe. For the severe ones — when you've broken a limb, severely bruised an area, or torn a muscle fiber, tendon, or ligament — you need to see a doctor immediately. He or she will treat your specific injury to enable it to heal properly. Many severe injuries require surgery, casts, medication, and rest. All painful injuries should be treated by a physician. After that, the information here may assist you in recovering the use of your injured part and preventing further injury.

Movement can be healing, if not for your injured part, then for the parts nearby and for the rest of your body. Although your doctor may not be familiar with the details of the many rehabilitative programs now available and therefore may not wish to recommend a specific rehabilitative regime, most doctors would agree that you should, if at all possible, maintain modified activity in order to stay in shape while the injury is healing.

*

Principles of Special Care

Listen, balance, revise, and stop — this summarizes the principles for you to follow to maintain, renew, and rehabilitate your body.

(1) *Listen* to the messages your body sends you, because in most cases they are the most important cues for body preservation. The first message you need to listen to is pain. Pain can actually be your friend. When some part of your body sends you a pain message, you should stop what you are doing and either adjust your activity to eliminate the pain or stop the activity altogether. The other messages you need to listen to are the sensations of warmth and fatigue you experience when you are safely strengthening, and the relaxing and softening sensations you feel from muscles safely stretching. And last, when you are doing vigorous activity or aerobic exercise you feel no sensation except the exertion of moving — no pain, no strong stretching, and no burning strengthening sensations.

2. *Balance* the use of your muscles. If your muscles have been contracting, then you need to stretch them, and if your muscles have been stretching, then you need to carefully strengthen them. By having your muscles in a state of pliable readiness, you can enjoy physical activity without worrying about injuring yourself. And after injury, if you balance strengthening activity with stretching exercises, you can help eliminate pain and get back to your activities sooner.

3. *Revise* your old habits of work, play, and even rest, if necessary, to be mechanically sound. Throughout this chapter you'll find guidelines for adjusting the mechanical ways you use your body. These small adjustments can make a big difference in helping you maintain your body in top condition.

4. *Stop* each day and take the time to rehabilitate your body. Stop your daily activities to do your stretching and strengthening exercises. Commit a small amount of time each day to special care of your body. Then relax and enjoy your investment in yourself. Be sure to relax. Let self-care be a habit.

Your Special Body

You have a very special body and it is the only one you'll get. You inherit your structure just the way you inherit your eye color and right- or left-handedness. Your joint structure contributes to your ability to coordinate your body. If you have loose ligaments, you are more prone to injury and have a harder time stretching your muscles. If your joints are tight, then you are less likely to have severe injuries but you are prone to muscle tears if you do not stretch your muscles properly and adequately.

How you use your body every day also contributes to the state of your muscles. Your level of physical activity, the nature of your work — sedentary, moving, passive, or active, your recreational and rest activities, and even the kind of bed and pillow you use will affect your body's condition. You need to keep all these factors in mind when you take special care of yourself.

UNEVEN LEG LENGTH

Everyone has a shorter leg. You know that one of your feet is bigger than the other. And you know that one of your hands is bigger than the other: when you wear tight-fitting gloves, you can feel the difference in the size of your hands. Some women know that one ear is lower than the other because one earring hangs lower than the other. And you know that one side of your face is not exactly the same as the other. In other words, you know that your body is not perfectly symmetrical. Compensating for your uneven leg length can correct many of the mechanical causes of pain and injury and help prevent an injury from recurring. You may not know that one of your legs is about ¼ to ⅜ of an inch longer than the other. Some people have a ½-inch difference! In any case, wearing a heel cushion the proper height under the heel of your shorter leg can relieve the mechanical stress in your neck, shoulder, upper back, lower back, hip socket, knee, and ankle.

If you have no pain, problem, or disability, should you

measure your legs and wear a heel lift? This is entirely up to you. Some back specialists feel that most back pain can be prevented this way, and others completely disagree. I believe in wearing a heel lift to prevent uneven use of all parts of your body and to act as a deterrent against injury. It is a painless precaution you can take, and it is your choice.

There are several ways to measure your legs. Some of them you can do by yourself and for others you'll need help. To measure your legs yourself, look in the mirror and see if one hip is higher than the other. That is the clearest sign that one of your legs is longer. See if the opposite shoulder is lower. If it is you have a *C* curve in your spine. (Everyone has either a *C* or an *S* curve.) If your shoulder is lower on the same side as your higher hip, then you have an *S* curve. See if your knees are the same height. See if the higher knee is on the same side as your higher hip. (That information may or may not help you find your short leg.) Or you can use a carpenter's level to find which leg is shorter. Stand on a firm floor, not a soft rug, with your feet together and put a sturdy belt around your hips. Place a carpenter's level on your belt. Often you will see the bubble in the level go up toward your long leg. Place a heel lift of approximately ¼ to ⅜ inch under your short leg and the bubble will move to the middle of the level.

To have someone else measure your leg, you will need a cloth or plastic tape measure. Lie on your back, with your shoes off. On each side of the front of your hip bone you will find a place where the bone has a corner. That is, the bone curves horizontally around your waist toward your belly button and then turns a corner and goes straight down toward your legs. Place your second finger on that spot on each side. This is where the person who is measuring your legs needs to start the tape measure on each side. Have your friend kneel down and place one end of the tape measure at the spot your finger is marking on your hip bone, and then stretch the tape down to the inside of your ankle where you have a small round bone that sticks out, *XVI-1*. Your friend should find the bottom of that round bone and push in on your foot so you can feel the end place being measured.

Next have your friend walk around to the other side of you and do this measuring on your other side. Walking around

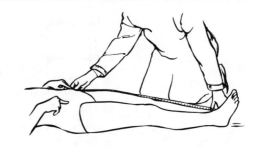

XVI-1

to your other side is necessary because if your friend reaches across you he or she may handle the tape differently, *XVI-2.* If the difference between your legs is not apparent after this first attempt to measure, then repeat the process and make sure that the tape starts at the same place on your hip bone and ends at the same place under your ankle bone. Then stand up and let your friend press down on your hip bones at your waist, to feel if one of your hips is higher. Then slide something under your short leg that is the height of the unevenness of your legs, such as pages of a book or magazine. Then have your friend press down on your hip bone as before and see if the unevenness is corrected. You will feel the difference with the heel lift under your short leg. Stand there 30 seconds to a minute. Then step down and feel the difference. You may feel as though you stepped into a hole. Then step back on the heel lift and feel your shoulder, neck, and back rearrange slightly. Some people with back pain feel the difference immediately. There is a softening of a specific tension in the area of stress from the uneven mechanical strain.

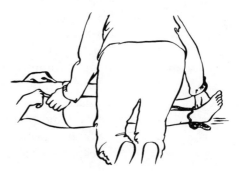

XVI-2

Get a bunch of correct-height heel cushions and put one in every shoe of your short leg. Put one in your bedroom slipper, your hiking boot, your ice or roller skate, your ski boot. If the heel cushion is uncomfortable inside your shoe, then have a shoemaker attach one to the bottom of the heel of your shoe.

Sometimes sitting on a cushion the height of your heel cushion helps prevent spasm. If you have a *C* curve in your spine, then put the cushion under the sitz bone of your short leg. If you have an *S* curve, put it under the sitz bone of your long leg. Try this and see if you get comfort in your upper body. If you don't, then use only the heel cushion and don't bother with the sitz bone cushion.

The following problems are often connected to and, in part, derived from uneven leg length: sore neck, sore shoulder, sore back, sore buttock, clicking hip, and pain in the groin. Here are some suggestions for what you can do about these problems.

SORE NECK

Though you can overdo many different activities and wake up the next day with a sore neck, or what people call a "crick" in the neck, there are some preventative mechanical actions to take to lessen your soreness. The first is to have your legs measured and wear a heel lift under your short leg. Most often the soreness is on the short-leg side.

The second is to sleep (when you sleep on your side) with pillows the height of your ear to the edge of your shoulder. Your pillow or pillows should be high enough to keep your spine in a gentle straight line, to prevent it from bending or twisting, which happens when you lie on your side with the wrong pillow or none. Then you will not need to cram your bent arm under a too-low pillow to lift your head up to a more comfortable height. The tension from sleeping with your arm in that position contributes to your neck soreness. You don't need to run out to buy new pillows. Fold a big towel and place it under the pillow you already use to give you the specific height you need. Another mechanical aid for resting comfortably is a rolled towel put under your waist when you sleep on your side. Roll it only to the thickness that fits your body. These two aids allow your spine to rest in a straight line and feel very good!

Do the following exercises to help a sore neck: First do Snow Angel and Hug the World (exercises 13 and 14). Then do Shoulder Stretches from below, the side and above (exercises 10–12). Then carefully do the Neck Stretches to the center, side, and diagonal (exercises 1–3). Then do Head Raises, center, diagonal, and side and rotating (exercises 4,5,7). Repeat the neck stretches after completing the strengthening ones. Usually after completing this series of exercises, you should feel much less soreness in your neck. Often it is possible to eliminate it completely.

Keeping your head in correct alignment is a worthwhile measure to take to prevent a sore neck. When your head slides forward and you carry it that way, your neck muscles have about 40 pounds of drag on them instead of balancing the usual 10- to 12-pound weight of your head. That is, the weight of your head is four times its normal weight when it is not aligned with your ears above your shoulders. This forward-head position results in pain under the top inside area of your shoulder blades.

SORE SHOULDER

There are two common places of soreness in the shoulder. One is discussed above and is caused by forward head carriage. The second occurs directly at the shoulder joint. This pain is an example of "point" pain rather than surface pain. The discomfort is right where your bones come together: they feel as though they are not in the right place, which is often the case. When your shoulder blade slides too far forward, the part of that bone that is connected to your collarbone (these two bones make up the top part of the shoulder joint) presses on the ligament, which in turn becomes swollen. This swelling presses on the bursa (bursae are little sacs in all your joints, which release fluid in response to irritation). The bursa can then become inflamed and press on the nerve. And that hurts.

If you carry your shoulder blade down and back (see Alignment [exercise 98]), you will prevent this injury. If you reposition your shoulder when you feel pain there, you can relieve some of the pain right away. That is the major mechanical change you need to make. It follows that you should learn to carry your shoulder blades in the correct position. And guess what? This injury often occurs on the side of your short leg; so make sure to measure your legs and wear your heel cushion. Also, sitting on a sitz bone cushion may help.

To balance your muscles so that the ones in front of your shoulders are less tight and the ones in back are stronger and less stretched, do the following exercises: Snow Angel (exercise 13); shoulder stretches from below, the side, and above (exercises 10–12); neck stretches and strengthening (exercises 1–5); then Hug the World (exercise 14), Chicken (exercise 15) with weights, and Side Wall Push-ups (exercise 29).

SORE BACK

Book after book has been written about how to handle back pain and injury. After reading the anatomy section of Chapter 10, you should know why there is so much written on the subject. Since it is very difficult to actually strengthen your back, you always need to guard against back injury. But there are things you can do to help you live through back pain until it goes away, which it eventually does.

There are several mechanical adjustments you can make for your back. Some of the most important ones have been described in the sections on Uneven Leg Length and Sore Neck, above. You need to have your legs measured and wear a heel lift. When you sleep on your side, you need pillows the height of your ear to the edge of your shoulder, a rolled towel under your waist, a 3- to 4-inch pillow to put between your knees, *XVI-3*. If you need to sleep on your stomach, then put a pillow under your stomach area and don't use a pillow for your head. If you sleep on your back, use a very low pillow for your head and pillows under your legs.

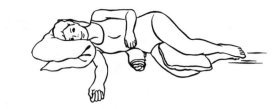

XVI-3

When you have severe back pain, you may wish to spend most of the night in the Super Back Rest position (exercise 51). The pillows under your legs should be the height of your thighs. (Often your sofa cushions are useful here.) Your thigh and lower leg need to be at a right angle, and you should bend your knees toward your nose so that your thighs are at a greater-than-right angle. Put small pillows on each side of your head and none under, *XVI-4*, then when your head rolls sideways, it will be supported and you will not wake up with a sore neck.

When you sit, use a rolled towel behind and below your waist, and keep your spine aligned vertically. You may need to use a sitz bone cushion. (These suggestions may help you tolerate a ride in your car.) Put both your feet or one at a time up on a low stool. If you cross your legs, and it *is* all right to do that, you should keep changing your top leg. The slouch sitting position may feel good for a few minutes, but for a long time, it strains the ligaments in your spine and presses the disk fluid into too constricted a space, which may create another kind of soreness.

Wear low-heeled shoes, and if you stand a lot, stand with one foot forward or up on a little ledge, and keep changing

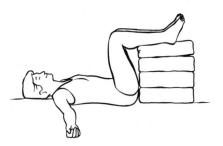

XVI-4

which leg is forward. Be sure to keep your knees unlocked! Unlocking your knees can relieve severe pain because then you can stand with your body correctly aligned.

You should do *all* the exercises in Chapter 10, "Your Lower Back and Hips." They work to relieve back pain and soreness and also to prevent it. You can do them as often as you need them. As a matter of fact, when you feel back pain start, don't let it remain in your body. Pull it out, using the Door Frame Pull (exercise 50), Open Tailor Sit (exercise 54), Super Back Rest (exercise 51), or any of the others in Chapter 10. And when you are up to it, start strengthening your abdominal muscles with Curl-downs (exercise 47) or Pussy Cat and Leg-Arm-Head Lifts (exercises 45, 46). Strong abdominal muscles do not guarantee that you won't hurt your back, but they can make your back less vulnerable.

The tighter the muscles on the back of your legs, the more likely your back pain will persist. So you need to use the following stretches to handle that part of your back care. Make sure to do calf stretches and probably the Phone Book Calf Stretch (exercise 88); the Triple Hamstring Stretch (probably just the one lying on the floor while your back heals); the Sitting Quadriceps Stretch (exercise 61); and the Pretzel (exercise 56). These next suggestions seem very simple but they are *very important!* If you do the hamstring stretch standing, make sure to have your heel cushion under your short leg. When you do the Pretzel, be sure to sit on your sitz bone cushion. These simple devices can keep muscle spasms from occurring when you do these exercises.

SORE BUTTOCK OR "SCIATICA"

Soreness in the hip may be deep in your buttock, producing radiating pain or numbness around and down into the front of your thigh, as in sciatica; or it may occur in the socket and only hurt when your leg is in some positions. The first kind of pain is most often on your long-leg side, the other can be on either side. Have your legs measured and put a heel lift in the shoe of your short leg. When sitting, you may find comfort from a sitz bone cushion. Correct alignment helps, especially unlocking your knees.

The major exercise that relieves this pain is the Open Tailor Sit (exercise 54), but don't do it until you have done a quadriceps stretch (exercises 61–65), a Pretzel (exercise 56), and a hamstring stretch (exercise 71). Some strengthening exercises tire the spasming muscles, and the Open Tailor Sit relieves the soreness more completely. Side-thigh strengthening (exercises 71, 78) and Leg-Arm-Head Lifts (exercise 46) work well to tire the group of muscles you need to stretch. The Chiropractic Position (exercise 53) also helps pull out the sore muscles. Follow all the guidelines in the Sore Back section above.

Soreness inside the joint often occurs if you have loose ligaments. Your quadriceps muscles need extra stretching and you need to use the loose ligament quadriceps stretch and Deep Lunge (exercises 65, 66) before you will be able to do the Pretzel or Open Tailor Sit with comfort in that joint. Sometimes placing a shoe or rolled towel under the thigh of the sore hip socket lets you bend your upper body forward without that point pain.

CLICKING IN THE HIP SOCKET

The sensation of something rubbing and rolling over something deep inside your hip joint with an accompanying sound when you do Leg Extensions (exercise 68) is described variously as "clicking" or "popping." The sensation is unpleasant; you can feel it about to happen, and you often get relief when it is done. It comes from ligaments or tendons rolling over each other, and it is preventable. (It occurs in your neck, ankles, and hands, too.) Sometimes moving more slowly helps prevent it. Using a heel lift also keeps your body aligned correctly and can prevent it in your neck. When it occurs in your legs, it is most often on your long-leg side.

To prevent clicking in your hip when you do Leg Extensions: (1) don't "turn out" your leg quite so much. Then (2) relax your hip, at your waist, so it is level with your other one. **(3)** Try to extend your spine upward by trying to touch your head to the ceiling and actively hold in your abdominal muscles. **(4)** Transfer your weight farther forward on your standing foot, because if you are standing too far back the leg muscles on the front and back of your leg can't work evenly. This last guideline may be the most helpful. As you lift and lower your leg **(5)** keep your muscles relaxed and don't grab with them. **(6)** Make sure that your foot is aligned straight out from your ankle. This fine adjustment helps distribute the weight of your leg evenly on your thigh muscles.

PAIN IN THE GROIN

This kind of pain is a specific, "point," pain and not the kind of pain that comes from a pulled or torn muscle, though it may feel like it. If you try stretching out this discomfort using the Three-Part Inner Thigh Stretch (exercise 76) and that only seems to help temporarily, you should check the heels of your shoes, and especially your running shoes, if you run. Your heels may be worn down a lot and need replacing. The wear may be more on the shoe of your short leg than on the shoe of your long leg, and the pain in your groin be more (or only) on the side of your short leg. Replacing your worn heel, or your shoes, if necessary, should eliminate the pain. Of course, <u>make sure you are walking and running with your feet and knees straight ahead</u>.

The Deep Lunge stretch (exercise 66) may also help to pull out the discomfort. After you stretch your leg straight back, and with your hip turned down toward the floor, turn your foot so your heel is in and not out, as it is in the second part of the stretch. This new foot position will let you stretch the inside of your thigh and help relieve the pain in your groin. {**Troubleshooting:** Be very careful to keep your knee straight but not locked in this turned-out position. Also be sure not to bend it when you are stretching in this position, because your knee is in a very vulnerable position.} The results of this stretch also may be only temporary. You will need to even out your shoe heels to prevent the pain from recurring.

The *Stretch and Strengthen* Method of Special Care

The approach to handling injury presented here involves working with muscles and mechanics. What does that mean? Pain comes from trauma to a part of your body and it also comes from muscle spasms that result from your body's response to that trauma. By carefully stretching muscles in the area of your pain, you can pull out the muscle spasms and that greatly helps to relieve pain. When a body part is not in its mechanically correct position, that can cause you to use that part in a faulty way, which can contribute to your pain. When you put that part in its correct place and stretch and strengthen your muscles so that that part can remain in its correct place, then you can markedly lessen your pain.

This approach to handling injury seeks to find the mechanical *cause* of your injury and *prevent* it from happening again by suggesting ways for you to relearn the habits of moving so you can use your limbs in a mechanically advantageous manner. Much of the information here uses the basic principles of body mechanics that have been taught for years. However, you are more likely to pay attention to these principles when you are trying to get rid of pain and get back to enjoying your favorite activity.

TENNIS ELBOW

Tennis elbow even happens to people who don't play tennis. Soreness occurs in the elbow joint's tendons and ligaments as well as lower in the forearm. You can feel discomfort from this injury above and below its site. Sometimes tingling occurs down the forearm and into your ring and little fingers.

Here are the mechanical adjustments to make: Have your legs measured and wear a heel cushion. Carry your head correctly aligned. For tennis, wrap your tennis racket handle with a thick layer of foam rubber so you can't grip the handle quite so hard. Do this for anything else you have to grip or carry. When possible, use bags with shoulder straps to carry your belongings. Be sure your shoulder blades are correctly aligned. Keep your elbow down as you lift and swing the racket — not out, sideways.

You need to do the same exercises as for people who have a sore shoulder (see above). Then you need to do the Wrist Stretch and Wrist Circles (exercises 21, 33) in as many hand and starting positions as you have patience for. Also do the Finger Circles, Finger Presses, and Slow Piano Playing (exercises 36–38). Musicians who have this problem don't need finger strengthening, but you do need the finger stretches that you get in Wrist Stretch.

STITCH IN THE RIBS WHEN RUNNING

This discomfort can be relieved even while you are running. Stretch up your waist, and then use the Shoulder Stretch from Below (exercise 10). Try to stretch one side, then the other, before you stretch both sides. You may only need to stretch the side on which you have the stitch. Put that shoulder up and the other shoulder down. After you complete this stretch and have pulled out the discomfort, make sure that your head is aligned correctly and that your chin is in.

SORE KNEES

You can feel sore knees deep inside, under your knee cap. This condition is often called chondromalacia. You also feel soreness on the inner and outer sides of your knees. Unlocking your knees helps relieve pain in all three areas, and it is very important to learn to do this all the time. Have your legs measured and wear a heel lift under the heel of your short leg. Walking correctly will also help you eliminate pain. Place each foot straight ahead, press your toes down on each step, and be sure that your knee goes directly over your foot and does not wander in or out on any part of your walk. If you can't find someone to watch you walk, then walk toward a full-length mirror and watch to see if your knees stay directly over your feet.

The exercises that your leg muscles need are the following: all three calf stretches and probably the Phone Book Calf Stretch (exercises 84–88); the hamstring stretches (exercises 71, 72); the quadriceps stretches (exercises 61–65); and the Pretzel (exercise 56). You may need to do Parentheses (exercise 82) to train your knees to go straight over your feet. You'll need Ankle Crisscross and Sand Scraping (exercises 91, 92) for your ankles, and the Inchworm and Hiccup (exercises 95, 97) for your toes.

PAIN BEHIND THE KNEES WHEN STRETCHING

If you feel pain behind your knees when you do calf stretches, hamstring stretches, or the Three-Part Straddle Stretch, then you have received a very important signal that you have extra-tight calf muscles and need to do the Phone Book Calf Stretch (exercise 88). When you are doing these other stretches, there are a few adjustments you can make for your legs to eliminate the pain. For calf stretches only use positions in which you actually feel stretching in your muscles. While you do the Standing Hamstring Stretch (exercise 71), put a small book ¾ to 2 inches high under your heels so you can feel the stretch in the backs of your thighs and not have any pain in the backs of your knees. When you are doing the Three-Part Straddle Stretch (exercise 79), put a rolled towel under your knees, or use anything soft that is high enough to support your knees while you stretch. That support should enable you to feel the stretching in your muscles and not under your knees. This pain will diminish entirely as you adequately and safely stretch your muscles.

MUSCLE CRAMPS

The most common cramps occur in your calf muscles and toes. A cramp is a contraction that won't relax. You need to know only one main thing to take out muscle cramps: If you *bear weight on that body part,* the opposite set of muscles will take over to help release the cramp. Here are some specific examples: When you are swimming and your calf muscle cramps, get out of the water and stand on the foot of the leg that is cramping and bend your knee. Stay in that position until you feel the cramp relax. When your toes cramp at night, get up and stand on the ball of your foot, on tiptoe, until you feel your cramp let go.

The common way to handle a cramp is to knead it with your hands. That takes much longer and may not always work. The result may be that your muscle is very sore after the cramp because it lasted so long. You should consider stretching these cramping muscles before you do your activity, even stretching your leg and feet muscles before you go to sleep.

Cramps may come from a sodium and/or potassium imbalance in your blood stream. They may also come from a lack of calcium absorbed in your body. Some people get leg and toe cramps after riding on a bicycle seat that presses too deeply into the groin. These causes should be considered along with very tight muscles. Nevertheless, the most effective way to relieve a cramp is to bear weight on it.

SORE LEG MUSCLES

You can have sore leg muscles from bouncing your stretches instead of holding them. You may also have pulled or torn a muscle during activity or doing improper readying exercises. Torn muscles have a more specific pain location and eventually a bruised area emerges under your skin. Pulled muscles are just very sore but do not have the characteristics of a torn muscle.

Here are basic guidelines for the care of sore and injured muscles.

- Check with a doctor to make sure no bone is broken and no ligaments or tendons are torn.

- Let the injury heal for 3 to 5 days. Do not do any activity with the injured part for 3 to 5 days, or until you no longer feel "Ouch!" pain in that area.
- If possible, stretch the muscles near and around the injury to prevent stiffness.

• Resume gentle and modified activity when the pain is gone.

Most professional sports people, dancers, and circus performers keep in action in spite of this kind of pain. One of the best ways to keep going is to gently and carefully stretch out the muscles of the injured area. Then you can keep your leg moving and thereby diminish the pain because the fluid that comes into the area that causes it to swell up (to bring the protein to heal the injury) keeps circulating and moves out of the area. This reduces the swelling, markedly lessens the pain, and prevents stiffness which can, at times, be just as painful as the injury.

You should do your stretching in a warm bath or shower or when your muscles are literally very warm. If you are outside, make sure to have layers of warm clothing on your legs. You will need to take much longer to stretch the leg that has a pulled muscle or muscle tear. The extra time is well worth it because you won't lose days of activity. It only takes minutes to give extra care to your muscles. Don't resume your full, all-out activity until your soreness has lessened enough for you to walk comfortably. During this 24- to 48-hour period, keep moving, because your moving will keep your muscles in tone and prevent the injured area from becoming stiff.

All the mechanical corrections for standing, walking, and running are useful here, because you will be more able to maintain your activity level if your joints are without mechanical stress from misuse.

SORE ACHILLES TENDONS AND CALF MUSCLES

An inflamed Achilles tendon, or tendinitis, is a common injury among active people. This diagnosis refers to an inflammation of the tendon that attaches your calf muscles to the base of your heel. Sometimes the tendon itself feels sore, and sometimes the area in front of your tendon and even on both sides of your ankle is sore. It is important to pay attention to this pain. You want to eliminate it to prevent the possibility of your tendon's eventually rupturing.

The mechanical corrections are simple and similar to those listed above for sore knees. Have your legs measured and wear a heel lift under the heel of your short leg. While your tendon hurts, it may help to lift both of your heels ¼ to ½ inch to take a little stress off the bases of your tendons. Don't do any activity that makes you feel any discomfort. The soreness must heal. Correct walking techniques are important. Shorten your stride by about 1 to 2 inches so each step will produce a little less stress on your heels. Make sure to use your toes, which will enable you to extend your ankle on the push part of each step.

For your muscles, you must do the Phone Book Calf Stretch (exercise 88). Before you do this stretch do the Ankle Crisscross and Sand Scraping (exercises 91, 92) for your ankles, and the Inchworm (exercise 95) for your toes. Don't feel the calf stretch in your tendon; keep the stretching sensation in your calf muscles. This injury will heal, but you must give it all the time it needs.

Many people who get tendinitis have extra-tight Achilles tendons. If your tendons are tight, you cannot bend your knees very deeply while standing on your feet. You may have trouble jumping very high. You probably don't feel Standing Calf Stretch (exercise 85) very much, and you cannot tolerate the severe stretch that you get from the A-frame Calf Stretch (exercise 87). You probably feel pain behind your knee when you do the Standing Hamstring Stretch (exercise 71). You must do the Phone Book Calf Stretch (exercise 88) to prevent tendinitis.

Not all people who get tendinitis have extra-tight Achilles tendons. Those of you with very loose ligaments may have trouble stretching your calf muscles, because your ankle ligaments are so loose that no standing angle is great enough to start stretching your calf muscles. In this situation, it is all right to stretch your heel down from a step. Make sure you are able to hold on to something firmly while you do this. Do this one foot at a time and hold the position for 30 seconds to a minute. If you have tendinitis, don't risk this extreme stretch, because it is too difficult to control the stretch and you don't want your foot to slip off the step or your tendon to rupture. Especially don't rise up and down quickly or even slowly while using a step to stretch your calf muscles, because you are giving your muscles two messages — stretch and contract — too close together. The little circuit breakers at the ends of your calf muscle fibers may send an overload signal and then you run the grave risk of rupturing that tendon.

SHIN SPLINTS

Many people who get shin splints have tight Achilles tendons, so you must follow the guidelines above. But shin splints primarily come from excess toe flexion. That means too much right-angle bend at the ankle. If you get shin splints, you probably walk without extending your ankle on each step and you don't use your toes to press down. Instead, you flex — lift up — your toes on each step. You can help take away the pain of shin splints on each step if you carry your foot forward relaxed and slightly extended at the ankle. When you are about to put it down on the ground, don't flex your toes up; keep them relaxed and ready to press down.

You also need to keep placing your feet straight ahead. Don't wear clogs of any kind, because to keep them on you need to keep your ankle flexed. If you extend your ankle, you will lose your shoe. Wearing clogs makes your shins more vulnerable to this painful injury.

If you got shin splints after doing a lot of jumping, you probably were not landing correctly. You need to land down to your heels and then bend your knees. If you land on straight legs, without bending your knees, you jar your lower leg and yank on the insertion of your toe muscles, which are attached to your shin. This is a major cause of shin splints.

SORE FEET

Sore feet usually means soreness on the bottoms of your feet and often under the balls of your feet. One foot may hurt more than the other. If your main arch hurts, you may be walking with your feet turned out instead of straight ahead. You need to walk with your feet pointing straight ahead. The more you press your toes, especially your big toe, the less pain you are likely to feel in your main arch. That is, your pain will diminish when you begin to use your toes, and you must also stop locking your knees. When you lock your knees, your ankles often roll in, and this action misaligns your ankle bones and stretches your main arch. So unlock your knees and press down your toes.

You need to do the Inchworm and Toe Curls and Uncurls (exercises 95, 93) for your toes, and the Ankle Crisscross and Sand Scraping (exercises 91, 92) for your ankles. When your toes are strong enough, then you might try Hiccup (exercise 97). Anytime you think of it, press down your toes and lift up the ball of your foot.

FALLEN METATARSAL ARCH

Severe and sharp pain under the ball of your foot is often caused by a "fallen" metatarsal arch. If you have a callous on the ball of your foot at the place between the base of your big toe and your next toe, you have a fallen metatarsal arch. The sharp pain is often directly under that callous. You need to press your toes down on every step. In order to gain strength in your toes to do this pressing, you need to do the Inchworm (exercise 95) as often as you can. That will strengthen your stretched muscles and keep your weight in front of the callous. By doing the Inchworm regularly, you probably can get rid of the callous in about six weeks, and if you press down your toes, you can markedly diminish your pain on each step. Only start to do the Toe Curl and Uncurl and Hiccup (exercises 93, 97) when you no longer feel pain under the metatarsal arch.

Correct walking and standing are important here, too. Keep your knees unlocked and your toes relaxed and not flexed as you carry your foot forward. Then press down with all five of your toes.

SORE TOES

Sore toes probably come from shoes that are too tight and don't allow your toes the proper amount of room. Baby shoes are the correct design because they have square toes. The big toe can reach straight ahead the way it is meant to reach. Adult shoes crowd toes. So first get shoes that allow your toes enough space sideways. During the summer, wear thongs as often as you can to help align your big toe. And you can even put little pieces of rubber between your big toe and the next to help your big toes reach forward instead of on a diagonal toward your other toes.

Do the Inchworm (exercise 95) as often as you can, to train your toes to work and to reach straight ahead. Also do Toe Open and Close (exercise 94). This may be very hard at first, so don't hesitate to use your hands to open your toes and then try to get your toe muscles to hold the position before they close again.

Hammer toes also develop because you don't have enough room in your shoes. The second toe will often contract if it is longer than your big toe and your shoes don't give it enough room. Try to stretch it as often as you can. Also do the Inchworm as often as you can and keep your contracting toe reaching out; don't let it fold at the knuckle. Use your fingers to help stretch out your bent toe and then try to keep your toe extended. At night, experiment with a soft wrap that holds it extended while you sleep. That will help stretch the ligament that is shortening.

*

After following these guidelines, you will become adept at using stretch and strengthening exercises to lessen pain, pull out muscle spasms, and prevent these kinds of injuries from occurring. Then by moving your muscles correctly, you will keep your muscles moving and that, after all, is your goal!

Bibliography

Alter, Judy. *Surviving Exercise.* Boston: Houghton Mifflin, 1983. (Six guidelines of safe exercise, chap. 2)

Anderson, J. E., M.D. *Grant's Atlas of Anatomy.* 8th ed. Baltimore: Williams and Wilkins, 1983. (For illustrations)

Bartenieff, Irmgard, with Lewis, Dori. *Body Movement, Coping with the Environment.* New York: Gordon and Breach, 1980. (Alignment, breathing, and whole body coordination, chap. 15)

Benson, Herbert, M.D. *The Relaxation Response.* New York: Avon, 1975. (Breathing, chap. 15)

Berry, William A. *Drawing the Human Form.* New York: Van Nostrand Reinhold, 1977. (For illustrations)

Brukett, Lee N. "Investigation into Hamstring Strains: The Case of the Hybrid Muscle," *Journal of Sports Medicine,* Sept./Oct. 1975. (Chaps. 11 and 12)

Cailliet, René, M.D. *Foot and Ankle Pain.* Philadelphia: F. A. Davis, 1968. (Chaps. 13 and 14)

————. *Knee Pain and Disability.* Philadelphia: F. A. Davis, 1973. (Chaps. 11 and 12)

————. *Low Back Pain Syndrome.* 3rd ed. Philadelphia: F. A. Davis, 1981. (Chap. 10)

————. *Neck and Arm Pain.* 2nd ed. Philadelphia: F. A. Davis, 1981. (Anatomy and injuries, chap. 4)

————. *Shoulder Pain.* 2nd ed. Philadelphia: F. A. Davis, 1981. (Chap. 5)

————. *Soft Tissue Pain and Disability.* Philadelphia: F. A. Davis, 1977. (Injuries to the neck and the other parts of the body, chap. 4)

Clarke, David H. *Exercise Physiology.* Englewood Cliffs, N.J., Prentice-Hall, 1975. (Warm-up, chap. 3)

Clarke, H. H. *Physical Fitness Research Digest,* series 6, no. 3. Washington, D.C.: President's Council on Physical Fitness and Sports, July 1976. (Abdominal exercises, chap. 9)

Craig, Timothy T., editor. *Comments in Sports Medicine.* Chicago: American Medical Association, 1973. (Problems of bouncing, introduction)

Cyriax, James. *Textbook of Orthopaedic Medicine.* 7th ed. London: Bailliere Tindall, 1978. (Chaps. 7 and 13)

de Lauteur, Barbara J. "Exercise for Strength and Endurance." In *Therapeutic Exercise.* 3rd ed. Edited by John V. Basmajian. Baltimore: Williams and Wilkins, 1978. (Chap. 2)

Drury, Blanche J. *Posture and Figure Control Through Physical Education.* Palo Alto, Calif.: Mayfield, 1970. (Exercises adapted and adjusted, chaps. 5 and 8)

Farfan, H. F. *Mechanical Disorders of the Low Back.* Philadelphia: Lea and Febiger, 1973. (Chap. 10)

Foster, Walter F. *Anatomy.* Tustin, Calif.: Walter Foster Art Books, 21, n.d. (For illustrations)

Gorman, David. *The Body Moveable, Blueprints of the Human Musculoskeletal System: Its Structure, Mechanics, Locomotor and Postural Functions.* 3 vols. Vancouver, B.C., Canada: Gorman, 1981. (Anatomy described throughout the book)

Grahame, R., M.D., and J. B. Jenkins, M.D. "Joint Hypermobility — Asset or Liability? A Study of Joint Mobility in Ballet Dancers." *Annals of Rheumatic Diseases* 31 (1972). (Chap. 1)

Halpern, Alan A., M.D. and Eugene E. Bleck, M.D. "Sit-up Exercises: An Electromyographic Study." *Clinical Orthopaedics and Related Research* 135 (1979). (Problem with traditional sit-ups, chap. 9)

Jacobson, Edmund, M.D. *You Must Relax.* New York: McGraw-Hill, 1962. (Relaxation technique, chap. 1)

Jones, Kenneth G., M.D. "The Unstable Knee of the Young Athlete." *Journal of Arkansas Medical Society* 72, no. 11 (April 1976). (Chaps. 11 and 12)

Keller, Richard H., M.D. "Traumatic Displacement of the Cartilagenous Vertebral Rim: A Sign of Intervertebral Disk Prolapse." *Radiology* 110 (January/March 1974). (Chap. 10)

Kendall, Henry O., and Florence P. Kendall. *Muscles: Testing and Functioning.* Baltimore: Williams and Wilkins, 1949. (Explanations of terms used throughout the book)

Kendall, Henry O., Florence P. Kendall, and Dorothy A. Boynton. *Posture and Pain.* 4th ed. Baltimore: Williams and Wilkins, 1952. (Alignment, chap. 15)

Knott, Margaret, and Dorothy E. Voss. *Proprioceptive Neuromuscular Facilitation: Patterns and Techniques.* 2nd ed. Philadelphia: Harper & Row, 1968. (Chap. 2)

Lagerwerff, Ellen B., and Karen A. Perlroth. *Your Posture and Your Pains.* Garden City, N.Y.: Anchor Press/Doubleday, 1973. (Source of Inchworm, chap. 14)

Lichtor, Joseph, M.D. "The Loose-Jointed Athlete: Recognition and Treatment." *Journal of Sports Medicine* (Sept./Oct. 1972). (Chaps. 11 and 12)

McKenzie, Robin, M.N.Z.P., M.N.Z.T.A. *The Lumbar Spine: Mechanical Diagnosis and Therapy.* New Zealand: Spinal Publications, 1980. (Source of Floppy Push-ups, chap. 10)

Mensendieck, Bess M., M.D. *Look Better, Feel Better.* New York: Harper and Brothers, 1954. (Several exercises adapted, chap. 6)

Morehouse, Laurence E., and Leonard Gross. *Total Fitness in 30 Minutes a Week.* New York: Simon and Schuster, 1975. (Concepts of strength, chap. 2)

Nachemson, A. "The Load on Lumbar Discs in Different Positions of the Body." *Clinical Orthopaedics* 45 (1966). (Chap. 10)

Nicholas, James A. "Injuries to Knee Ligaments: Relationship to Looseness and Tightness in Football Players." *Journal of American Medical Association* 212 (June 29, 1970). (Chap. 1)

Noble, Elizabeth. *Essential Exercises for the Childbearing Year.* Boston: Houghton Mifflin, 1976. (Kegel Exercise, chap. 10)

Pansky, Ben. *Review of Gross Anatomy.* 4th ed. New York: Macmillan, 1979. (Anatomy, chap. 2)

Wells, Katherine F. *Kinesiology: The Scientific Bases of Human Motion.* 4th ed. Philadelphia: W. B. Saunders, 1978. (Explanations of several terms used throughout the book.)

Williams, Paul C., M.D. *Low Back and Neck Pain: Causes and Conservative Treatment.* Springfield, Ill.: Charles C. Thomas, 1974. (Neck and back injuries and exercises, chap. 4)

Index